Yoga
for a
Healthy
Lower
Back

*A Practical
Guide to
Developing
Strength and
Relieving
Pain*

Liz Owen *and*
Holly Lebowitz Rossi

Shambhala • *Boston & London* • 2013

This book is not intended to substitute for medical advice or treatment.

Shambhala Publications, Inc.
Horticultural Hall
300 Massachusetts Avenue
Boston, Massachusetts 02115
www.shambhala.com

Photos: ©Robert Zinck
Illustrations: ©Ann Boyajian
Chakra Symbols: (Illustration 16) ©Viktoriia Protsak—Fotolia.com

9 8 7 6 5 4 3 2 1

First Edition
Printed in the United States of America

♾ This edition is printed on acid-free paper that meets the
American National Standards Institute z39.48 Standard.
♻ This book is printed on 30% postconsumer recycled paper.
For more information please visit www.shambhala.com.
Distributed in the United States by Random House, Inc.,
and in Canada by Random House of Canada Ltd

Designed by James D. Skatges

Library of Congress Cataloging-in-Publication Data

Owen, Liz.
Yoga for a healthy lower back: a practical guide to developing strength
and relieving pain / Liz Owen, Holly Lebowitz Rossi.
pages cm
ISBN 978-1-61180-049-4 (pbk.)
1. Backache—Popular works. 2. Backache—Alternative treatment.
3. Yoga. I. Rossi, Holly Lebowitz. II. Title.
RD771.B217O94 2013
613.7'046—dc23
2013001181

For Ryah, *mija bonita,* and Peter Freeth Belford.
Los amo más de lo que la lengua pueda decir.   —L.O.

For Rob and Ben, with quiet prayers of thanks for the sunlight
each time I see your faces.   —H.L.R.

Contents

Acknowledgments

Gratitude can be such a powerful thing to feel but such a difficult a thing to express. Knowing that, we can only attempt to acknowledge, with grateful hearts, the broad community of mentors, experts, guides, resources, and friends who have been part of the process of creating this book.

Let's start at the beginning, when Steve Dyer designed our proposal with great skill and care. Raea Zani created a piece of art for the proposal that showed the sacrum in all its grace and glory. Susan Piver is not only an inspiring colleague and gifted writer but she was also kind enough to make our introductions at Shambhala, where Dave O'Neal took us in and put our project in the helpful, encouraging hands of Beth Frankl and Ben Gleason, who have guided us with great kindness and intelligence throughout this process.

The images you see throughout this book are the result of a great deal of work, planning, time, and, most important, artistry. Robert Zinck's photographic skills, equipment expertise, and time commitment—not to mention his yoga modeling—were invaluable. Thanks are due also to Shelley Zatsky for her photo-editing help that got us across the finish line. Christiana Melton not only modeled the yoga poses in this book with stunning beauty, she and her husband, Rex, allowed their home to be transformed into a photo studio on several occasions. We are also grateful to Chip Hartranft, of The Arlington Center, not only for founding the yoga studio where our personal and professional relationship was born but also for allowing us to shoot some of the book's photographs there. Finally, in the visual arts department, Ashley Lorenz and the Lilla Rogers Studio connected us with the gifted Ann Boyajian, whose exquisite anatomical illustrations have illuminated our text so beautifully.

Our book is greatly enriched by the experts we were fortunate enough to be able to consult for feedback and reactions. We are especially grateful to Jonathan Beasley of Harvard Divinity School for helping us find a Sanskrit consultant, and to Benjamin Williams for answering that call with such passion, enthusiasm, and intelligence. Chris C. Streeter, M.D., of Boston University School of Medicine, was so generous with her time and expertise in advising us on anatomy and Western medical concepts. We are also indebted to authors whose work has fueled and deepened ours, especially B.K.S. Iyengar, Edwin F. Bryant, Harish Johari, Vasant L. Lad and Anisha Durve, Thomas W. Myers, and Judith Hanson Lasater. Finally, a special OM to Georg Feuerstein, whose work was so valuable to us, and who passed away while we were working on this book.

Finally, some personal thanks from each of us.

From Holly: Thanks to Keith Puri of ChiroCare Associates for opening his bookshelf to us and for, together with Robert Kum, caring about my lower back all these years. Thanks are also due to Jill Feldman for her help with our contracts at the front end of this project. And gratitude of course to my family, especially Mom for being the first person to teach me about good posture; Dad for being my *consigliere* in all things; and my husband, Rob, and son, Ben, for keeping me upright in every sense of the word. This family list would not be complete without a note of thanks to my Gaga, Elaine Bassler Mardus, who sparked in me the curiosity and love of learning that inspired me to be a writer. Innumerable other friends and family members have offered their support, encouragement, and help in ways that are too great to list here. And finally, the most obvious but important thanks of all—to Liz Owen, an exceptional teacher and an exceptional person. My lower back has been transformed by my years in your class, and I'm so grateful that others will now get to learn from you, and from your yoga, as I have. I'm proud to stand beside you on this project.

From Liz: My first words of gratitude are to Holly Lebowitz Rossi, without whom this book would not have happened. The experience of collaborating with you, with your superb writing and editing expertise and your deep love and understanding of spirituality, religion, and yoga, is a true gift to me. I am so appreciative of your sure-footedness and graceful countenance, especially giving feedback on the first drafts. The going could have gotten rough, yet in your hands it was illuminative and joyful! From the day you said, "Let's write a book together," to the present, your congeniality has made our work flow more smoothly than I ever thought possible. I appreciate you so much.

To my longtime teacher and mentor, Patricia Walden, my heart is full of gratitude for your teachings, your insight, and your *prakasha*. There are so many yogis, alternative- and complementary-medicine practitioners, and others whose wisdom has infused my path with insight and inspiration through the years. Some of them are B.K.S. Iyengar, Karin Stephen, Zoe Stewart, Rod Stryker, Erich Schiffman, Gurmukh Kaur Khalsa, Dr. Ben E. Benjamin, Thich Nhat Hanh, Jon Kabat-Zinn, T.K.S. Desikachar, Paul Muller-Ortega, Ramanand Patel, Chip Hartranft, Richard Freeman, and Kit Laughlin. One thousand eight *namastes* to each of you.

To my family, I am ever grateful for the light you bring to my life. A huge thanks to all of you, and especially to Pete and Ryah for your patience during the writing of this book, and for understanding when I was basically a no-show everywhere but at my computer. To Vivian Everett, thank you for your encouragement and steadfast support—you always have my back. And to my amazing students, I am honored to share yoga—and life—with you. You bring me fullness and delight, and your bodies are *my* teachers, which constantly illuminate new insights and knowledge. This book would simply not be possible without you.

1

The Journey into Wellness

On this path effort never goes to waste, and there is no failure.
—the Bhagavad Gita

Your spine is one of the most physically important and symbolically powerful areas in your body. It is, after all, the column of support that holds you upright, enables you to stand tall, and connects your mind to your body.

Your lower back looms just as large, as the point from which you are rooted to the earth and stretch up toward the sky. Your lower back unites the two halves of your body; without it, you literally could not stand on your own two feet.

But let's face it—in modern American life, we hardly treat this complex, miraculous area with the respect it deserves. Ours is a culture of sitting for hours at a time, collapsing onto the couch at the end of a hard day, and accepting stress as both emotional and physical facts of daily life. Many of us work too hard, worry too much, and can barely find the time to visit our doctors to collect a diagnosis of "you work too hard and worry too much." Is it any wonder that lower back pain is an epidemic in America, the lower back acting like a beleaguered tagalong in the body rather than an open, flowing source of energy and activity?

I—for simplicity's sake, as coauthors we decided to use the first-person pronoun to represent Liz's voice throughout this book—believe the lower back is the most neglected area of the contemporary American body. But I also believe—and have seen during more than twenty years of teaching—that yoga is a healing path that can help relieve chronic lower back pain and build and sustain consistent lower back health.

This book is meant to meet you wherever you are in your journey toward health. If you have never practiced yoga before, you will find clear and accessible instruction to get you started. If you are an experienced yoga student but are wrestling with a lower back issue, you will find ways to bring what you know about yoga to fruition in your lower back . . . and progress into an even fuller, deeper practice.

Most of all, this book is meant to be an open dialogue with your body and what it's trying to tell you about what will help it heal.

JUST THE FACTS: YOUR BACK BODY

Reviewing some basic facts about your back and how it works (or how it can work) is the first step on your journey. Being educated about your basic anatomy is immensely helpful, both in identifying the sources and locations of your pain and in choosing poses and movements that bring relief and comfort to those areas.[1]

Your spine is divided into four main sections, each of which has a healthy, natural curvature (illustration 1). From top to bottom, they are:

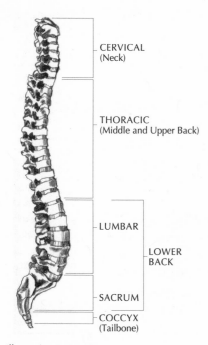

CERVICAL
(Neck)

THORACIC
(Middle and Upper Back)

LUMBAR

LOWER
BACK

SACRUM

COCCYX
(Tailbone)

Illustration 1. Your Spine

- Cervical spine—these seven vertebrae are at the top of your spine, at your neck. At their axis, the cervical spine connects your spine to your skull.
- Thoracic spine—these twelve vertebrae are your "middle and upper back" and they roughly cover the area behind your rib cage.
- Lumbar spine—these five vertebrae are where your "lower back" begins. Most of the movement your spine is capable of takes place in the lumbar area.

- Sacrum—these five vertebrae, which are fused together into a single bone, are at the very bottom of your lower back. Sacral health is crucial to the health of the entire spine, and because of this, and because of the sacral bone's distinctive shape, I call it "the heart of the spine."

Below the sacrum is your coccyx, often referred to as your "tailbone." There are four tiny, fused vertebrae that make up this bony area.

You know your back is capable of movement, but did you know that there are six distinct ways your back can move? We work with all of these in yoga:

- Flexion, otherwise known as forward bending
- Extension, or back bending
- Lateral movement, or bending to the side, either right or left
- Twisting, which can also be done either to the right or left

There are a few more terms you should learn, because they're referenced often throughout this book. The first is *myofascia*. The dictionary defines *fascia* as "a sheet of connective tissue covering or binding together body structures."[2] *Myo-* is a prefix used in medical jargon to denote that something has a relationship to muscle.[3] Thus, myofascia is the connective tissue that binds muscles together. Myofascia is crucially important in the process of opening your body by stretching; if your myofascia is tight, it will prevent the muscles it's connected to from lengthening and receiving the fresh, oxygenated blood they crave.

In medical and anatomy texts, the word *myofascia* is usually used when describing the function of an individual muscle and its surrounding and embedded connective tissues. Because yoga is a holistic practice, I think of myofascia as a continuous web of connective tissues and muscles through which the entire body acts, moves, and interacts among its various parts.[4]

A few more terms to review: a *tendon* is a band of dense, fibrous connective tissue that connects muscle to bone and distributes the force that muscle exerts,[5] and for simplicity's sake, it is considered in this book to be part of the myofascial web. A *ligament* is a fibrous band of tissue connecting bone to bone or supporting an organ in place.[6] You'll see that ligaments are noted throughout the book as distinct from myofascia, because they relate to bones rather than muscles.

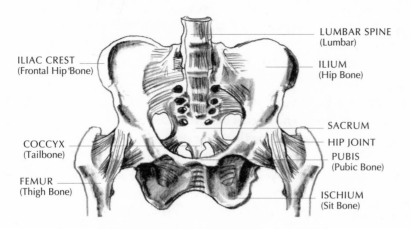

ILIAC CREST
(Frontal Hip Bone)

LUMBAR SPINE
(Lumbar)

ILIUM
(Hip Bone)

SACRUM

HIP JOINT

COCCYX
(Tailbone)

PUBIS
(Pubic Bone)

FEMUR
(Thigh Bone)

ISCHIUM
(Sit Bone)

Illustration 2. Your Lower Back and Hips

From right where you're sitting, it's easy to feel how the parts of your body are connected in the holistic view I'm referring to as the myofascial "web"—just reach your right arm up over your head and stretch it over to the left as you lean slightly to the left in your chair. You should feel a stretch not only in your right arm, but also along your right armpit and the side of your trunk, maybe all the way down to your waist.

You'll experience the connectedness of your entire body as you practice the yoga poses in the book, feeling how a particular stretch or movement travels through you. And you will come to understand how movement, or tightness and tension, in one part of your spine affects its other parts. You'll come to see your spine as an organic whole, and to appreciate the role that your lower back plays within it.

Your lower back, as we're addressing it in this book, consists of two major parts: your sacrum and your lumbar spine. We will also work with the lower back's immediate neighbors, your hips and abdominal core, because these areas are all so connected. As illustration 2 shows, the skeletal outline of your lower back is what's known anatomically as "the pelvic girdle," plus the lumbar spine that rises out of it. Because this is not an academic text, you will notice terms like *hip bones* used throughout the book. The illustration shows the proper names of the bones and joints, as well as how I'll be referencing them. Please turn back to this page whenever you need to reacquaint yourself with this vocabulary, and reference this "cheat sheet" for reminders when you need them:

- Ilium: Hip bone
- Ischium: Sit bone
- Pubis: Pubic bone
- Sacrum: Sacral bone
- Iliac crest: Frontal hip bone
- Sacroiliac joint: Sacral joint (see also illustration 6)
- Coccyx: Tailbone
- Femur: Thigh bone

Physically speaking, the goal of yoga practice for a healthy lower back is to increase the tone of the body's muscles and the flexibility of its myofascia by moving the spine through its six directions of movement. In addition to increasing your body's ability to support itself, movement encourages the synovial membrane, an inner membrane of tissue that lines each of your joints, to secrete synovial fluid, which serves to lubricate your joints and help you move with increasing ease.[7]

If you opened this book because your lower back is achy, sensitive, or a chronic source of pain, you are far from alone. An estimated 80 percent of people will experience back pain during their lifetimes, and the most common complaint within this group is lower back pain.[8] Back pain is the most common musculoskeletal pain Americans bring to their doctors each year, and in the years 2002 to 2004, back pain came with a $30.3 billion price tag in direct health care costs.[9] Most lower back pain affects young and middle-aged adults, with eighteen- to sixty-four-year-olds making almost 75 percent of all health care visits for lower back pain in 2006, and it affects slightly more women (56 percent) than men.[10]

Lower back pain can take many forms, some clinically serious and others "just" due to everyday stress and strain. The high number of people who suffer from lower back pain points to the diversity of its causes and consequences. Although I believe yoga can bring healing to the lower back, either on its own or in combination with medical treatment, I must mention certain scenarios in which it's crucial you consult a doctor. These include:[11]

- If you have had strong, constant pain for two weeks or more
- If your pain is accompanied by a fever
- If your pain is the result of a traumatic incident, such as a fall or a car accident

NAME YOUR PAIN

When you go to the doctor with a lower back issue, it may be difficult to describe your pain. But being descriptive—even literary—can help your doctor start to decode what the source of your pain might be. Here are some words my students have used to describe their back pain over the years: *hot, lightning-like, dull, shooting, annoying, stabbing, spastic, angry, achy, throbbing, grippy, burning, sharp, jumpy, agonizing, awful, debilitating.*

- If you feel numbness or tingling for more than a few days
- If your pain gets worse at night, making sleep difficult or impossible

If you don't have any of the above issues but are not sure whether it is safe for you to begin a yoga practice, please consult your physician for confirmation. In the appendices at the back of this book, I have provided yoga sequences that are helpful for specific medical diagnoses, including herniated disks, sacral sprains, spinal stenosis, and spondylolisthesis. Wherever you are in your journey toward wellness, your practice is waiting for you!

Stress and Pain: The Relaxation Response

Often, your experience of pain has to do with much more than the physical architecture and injury history of your body. Stress manifests itself in physical ways as well as emotional ones, and pain is often the way it rears its ugly head. Whether you see stress as a cause of pain in itself, or as the cause of chronic muscle tension and poor posture that in turn causes your pain, there can be no doubt—stress is a guilty party in the story of lower back pain.

You have probably heard that yoga can help you manage stress, and that is very true. But there's nothing magical or mysterious about why the practice of yoga can have a calming, centering effect on your stress level. Yoga simply signals your body—specifically, your nervous system—to deploy its own method of regulating the effects of stress. In short, yoga helps your body activate its "relaxation response."

"The Relaxation Response" was named and made famous by Dr. Herbert Benson of Harvard Medical School in his groundbreaking 1975 book by the same name. The book is still in print today and has reportedly sold more than four million copies. Benson was one of the first scientists to clinically study stress as a physiological phenomenon, and mind-body practice as having physiological benefits. His research led him to conclude that conditions including anxiety, high blood pressure, hypertension, and headaches can be improved using meditation and other mind-body techniques.

These techniques aren't simple "feel good" practices, they actually have neurological benefit: they stimulate the parasympathetic nervous system (PNS), which is responsible for calming the muscles, slowing the heart rate, and generally keeping the body from overreacting to the stressors that surround it in everyday life. The PNS's partner, the sympathetic nervous system (SNS), is a far more jittery creature, responsible for the famous "fight or flight" response, or the survival instinct that gives us the burst of energy we need to escape from dangerous situations.

Of course, you have heard many times that the fight-or-flight response was designed to help our primitive ancestors escape from predators or invaders. It was not meant to be activated when the supermarket checkout line is longer than we anticipated, when our boss asks us to redo work we've spent hours on, or when we have a quarrel with a family member. In these modern-day stress scenarios, our biology can conspire against us—if our PNS isn't there to bring the SNS into balance. As Benson discovered, and as the vast field of complementary, or integrative, medicine accepts as its premise, mind-body work is a valuable and beneficial method of achieving this balance.

Benson notes a list of conditions that, when caused or affected by conditions like stress, can be improved using self-care techniques such as meditative yoga and deep breathing. You should be encouraged to learn that back and neck pain are included on this list.[12]

You won't likely be able to banish stress from your life altogether, but with the physical and energetic tools yoga has to offer, it is realistic to expect to be able to better manage your stress and, by extension, your pain.

How Yoga Can Help

Benson discovered in a scientific setting what yoga practitioners have known for centuries—yoga can calm and open the body in a way that allows it to release stress and pain, including, and especially for our purposes, lower back pain.

Yoga is—together with sitting meditation and a mindfulness technique called "body scan"—one of the three main components of the biologist Jon Kabat-Zinn's pioneering work with stress, pain, and illness.[13] Kabat-Zinn, working and teaching at the University of Massachusetts Medical School, created the Mindfulness-Based Stress Reduction (MBSR) program that is used in hospitals and pain clinics across the country. In his popular 1990 book *Full Catastrophe Living*, he calls yoga "another way in which you can learn about yourself and come to experience yourself as whole, regardless of your physical condition or level of 'fitness.'"[14]

Recent research supports what Benson, Kabat-Zinn, and many others have introduced to the mainstream. Study after study hypothesizes that your nervous system is directly affected by yoga practice.

I'll mention just one such study, a randomized controlled trial conducted in Boston and published in 2009. The study gave a twelve-week yoga course, including deep relaxation, yoga postures, and breathing techniques, to a group of people who were suffering from chronic lower back pain. At the end of the program, nearly three quarters of the participants reported a reduction of their pain; only 27 percent of the "control group," which had not been given yoga, reported similar improvement. Additionally, and remarkably, the participants who did the yoga program decreased their use of pain medications, reporting no usage at all of opiate analgesic medications by the end of the program.[15]

While all of the yoga in this book is an important part of the process of healing your lower back pain, I want to offer one more note about the ways *pranayama*, yogic breath work, can be a particularly healing practice, one that can soothe both your hurting body and your stressed mind. As you practice pranayama, please keep in mind everything you've learned about your PNS and SNS, and the power those systems have over your body's experience of stress and pain.

How does pranayama work on your nervous system? I'll give two quick examples. First, Three-Part Breath, or Dirgha Pranayama, which we'll practice on page 41, brings long, deep breaths into your pelvic area, abdomen, and chest. This sequential, mindful flow of breath not only releases muscle tightness in those areas, it also encourages the vagus nerve, which is responsible for stimulating the PNS, to send your heart relaxing messages through your long, deep exhalations. Second, in Ocean Breath (Ujjayi Pranayama, see page 12), even, elongated inhalations and exhalations are used to balance the SNS, which controls your body's fight-or-flight response to

THE SLOW ROAD, THE BEST ROAD

When I first began yoga, I studied with an exceptionally creative yoga teacher from California. He often started his workshops with seated poses, including Hero's Pose, in which you kneel, then sit back with your hips on the floor between your feet. Even though this is considered an appropriate pose for beginners, it can be quite challenging for students with tight thighs, hips, or ankles, or those with knee issues. The teacher had a trick to keep students from getting discouraged—he suggested we place a thick phone book under our hips to open our thighs and relieve pressure on our knees and ankles. Every day, he said, we were to remove one page in the phone book and practice the pose again. I did this, and indeed, at the end of a short three years (there were about 1,200 pages in the phone book I had), my hips were comfortably grounded on the floor in Hero's Pose. What's the moral of the story? First, *anything* can be a yoga prop . . . and second, patience leads to progress!

stress, and the PNS. When you make your exhalations longer than your inhalations in Ocean Breath, you stimulate the PNS even more deeply, eliciting the relaxation response.[16]

Finally, as you embark on your new yoga practice, let me share something that has been meaningful to me in my own yogic journey and that I will be using often in the yoga practice sections of this book. It's these three words: any amount possible!

"Any amount possible," said with quiet, focused gusto, is what echoes through my mind every time I practice yoga, especially when I am trying a challenging pose or working with a part of my body that is tight, stiff, or dull. It is an oft-used phrase from the Iyengar yoga tradition, the well-known alignment-based method of yoga founded by the living yoga master B.K.S. Iyengar.

These simple words were especially encouraging to me when I first started practicing yoga, because my body, and my lower back in particular, was very tight from years of hunching over a desk as an architect. Today, when I ask my students to stretch, reach, or open their bodies "any amount possible," I mean to remind them not to push their bodies beyond what they can comfortably and safely do at a given moment. Instead, I like to encourage them to create a dialogue with their bodies in order to understand how far they can move into a pose, and how much stronger and more flexible—even incrementally so!—they are becoming each time they are returning to a pose they have practiced before.

The words continue to inspire both my yoga practice and teaching today as I continually find more spaciousness and comfort in my own body and as I see those qualities develop in my students. On the physical level, the ability to meet your body where it is and ask it to open up any amount possible is one of the true gifts of yoga. I hope it can inspire you to practice so that you too will find renewed openness and strength in your own body.

What Is Yoga?

What are we to make of that fact that one person might practice yoga at a commercial gym in New York City, while another will travel to India to practice it with a renowned spiritual master? Or of the way one student might meditatively chant "om" with her hands pressed prayerfully together at the beginning of a yoga class, while another only looks forward to the physical rewards of a good, deep stretch?

Are both of these students—plus the estimated fifteen million Americans who practice yoga,[17] engaging in the same practice? In other words, what is "yoga"?

The answer is—like your body, like your life—not easy to simply or fully describe in a few paragraphs. It is, however, worthy of a few moments of contemplation; a fascinating amalgam of spirituality, physical fitness, and the intersection of ancient and contemporary culture.

Let's start with the meaning of the word itself. In Sanskrit, the language of ancient India, a prevalent meaning of *yoga* is "discipline," and the term can be used similarly to how we would describe broad academic categories—imagine "math yoga," "reading yoga," or "science yoga."

In the complex Indian religious tradition called Hinduism, which some scholars date as far back as 1500 B.C.E.,[18] there are at least five major "yogas," each of which is said to correspond to an aspect of the human personality: jnana yoga (discipline of knowledge), bhakti yoga (discipline of devotion), karma yoga (discipline of selfless action), raja yoga (royal discipline), and hatha yoga (discipline of physical exertion).[19]

It is this last yoga—hatha—that is most familiar to most of us as the disciplined use of bodily postures called asanas and breath work called pranayama. The term *yogi* or *yogini*, incidentally, is translated as "a man or woman of discipline."

There is a second, often-cited definition of the Sanskrit word *yoga*—"union." The word is related to the English word *yoke*, as in "to join."

Traditionally, the union yogis are pursuing is a spiritual one, between the Atman, which is loosely equivalent to the Western notion of the "soul" or "Self," takes toward Brahman, which can be defined as Absolute Being.

"Brahman" is an abstract idea in Hindu theology. The same Sanskrit root also forms the name Brahma, who is the divine creator and one of the three major deities, collectively referred to as the Trimurti, that make up the faith's core for some modern-day Hindus. (Vishnu, the Preserver, and Shiva, the Destroyer, are the other two.) In the most traditional sense of hatha yoga, its practitioners are calming, balancing, and strengthening their bodies for a purpose far beyond health or physical improvement—they are preparing their deepest selves for meditative union with the highest mystical consciousness.

In case you're starting to worry that this all sounds too "spiritual" or "out there" for you—or contrary to the teachings of your own faith—fear not. You do not have to practice Hinduism to practice yoga, and although the Westernization and secularization of yoga can be controversial in some circles, the fact remains that yoga shows up at practically every conceivable point along the spectrum of modern American life. *Yoga Journal's* 2008 "Yoga in America" study found, for example, that nearly half of Americans practice yoga for overall health, and nearly fourteen million Americans have had yoga recommended to them by doctors.[20]

So you can be assured that whatever your approach to your personal practice, the "discipline" and "union" of yoga can be as secular or as spiritual as is meaningful to you. It can simply be about releasing tension, pain, and imbalance in your body. It can be about quieting the chatter and fear in your mind so that your body can open up to greater health and wellness. You can imagine your practice as a way to bring into balance the multiple layers of yogic "bodies"—energetic, and mental or emotional among them—that are layered within your outermost, physical body.[21] Or you can envision your practice as a path toward what Patanjali, the compiler of the ancient treatise known as the Yoga Sutras, calls "meditative absorption" into a higher state of being.[22]

But one thing is certain, those two kinds of practitioners—one in a gym-based yoga class, the other at the feet of a master in India—are, in fact, both practicing yoga. And in your journey through this book, you will discover your own path, your own discipline, your own yoga.

Of course, I haven't lost sight of the fact that you picked up this book because you are interested in how yoga can help you bring health, strength, and balance to your lower back. In yoga, everything is done with mindfulness and purpose, even the most basic, universal human actions. We'll start our journey by exploring yogic insights on four of these: breathing, standing, sitting, and resting.

How to Breathe

"Just breathe." It's what you might say to a friend who is talking a mile a minute to bring you up to speed on a personal crisis. It's what you might have been told to do when the stresses of your life have put you off your game. And it's what you often likely murmur to yourself when you're experiencing back pain, whether chronic or acute.

Breath, as you know, is the life-giver and sustainer, one of the most powerful symbols of our constant connection to the basic, miraculous fact that we are alive. Yet most of us go through each day without paying close attention to it at all. If we did, we would quickly realize that the quality, pace, and rhythm of our breath can be deciding factors in how smoothly any given day goes, and in how much more quickly we can move toward lower back health.

You'll encounter references to your breath often in this book, sometimes using the Sanskrit term *pranayama*, which means "breath control."[23] The reason for that is that breath work is a partner—many would say an equal partner—with physical postures in the practice of yoga. Your breath is a tool, to be used just as respectfully and mindfully as you would use your muscles, your bones, or your brain. But like all tools, you must learn *how* to use it if you are going to experience its full power.

Generally speaking, when you practice yoga poses (asanas), your breath should be full, smooth, and rhythmic, taking as long to inhale as you do to exhale. In my classes, I advise students to use their breath this way: "A strong breath for a strong pose, a soft breath for a soft pose." That means that when you are practicing a pose that takes a lot of energy, such as a standing pose or a backbend, you should breathe very deeply—ideally, in a softly audible way—to help your body move into the pose, to support your body while you are in the pose, and to help you to come out of it. Remain mindful of your breath, especially in challenging poses, because you may discover a tendency to hold it when your body is working hard. When that happens, gently bring your breath back into your body with a deep, even, audible inhalation and exhalation—you'll feel a big, immediate difference in how you experience the pose. Remember, though, when you are in a restful or meditative position, to let your breath become soft and quiet, encouraging your body and mind to relax.

When you focus your mind on your breath as well as on your body, your mind is drawn inward. It learns to observe, witness, and become present to the sensations in your body—especially, for our purposes, the critical messages your lower back is trying to tell you about its condition and what will help it to come into wellness. A natural, full flow of breath can help to open tight areas, release tension, and bring life force (prana) into its full expression in your body.

The breath work (pranayama) exercises I will introduce in this book are meant to help you cope with chronic pain and the emotional stresses that come along with it. Much of the pranayama practice you'll learn in this book is meant to elicit the "relaxation response" I discussed earlier. When your emotions lose their charge and calm down, you can create a positive dialogue with your body and your pain, instead of living with the fear and anxiety that often accompany chronic pain. Remember, you can practice pranayama exercises whenever you feel pain or are mentally or emotionally charged or strained . . . and whether you're on and off your yoga mat. Once you connect with the power of your breath, you'll carry a self-sustaining treasure trove of wellness and life force wherever your life takes you.

Now let's learn one of the most powerful (yet accessible) pranayama practices I know of—Ocean Breath. You'll see this breath a number of times throughout this book, and I hope that it can become a go-to practice whenever you need to come into control of your breath and direct it toward your emotional or physical well-being.

Ocean Breath is called Ujjayi Pranayama in the yogic texts. *Ujjayi* means "upward victory," which is quite descriptive of how this breath feels and looks in your body, because when you practice it, your lungs are fully expanded and your chest lifts and broadens, like a mighty conqueror.[24] Yet the name Ocean Breath is lovely and apt as well, because as you will hear, it sounds like a gentle ocean wave breaking in the distance. You will create this sound by very slightly and gently narrowing the space between your vocal cords. Sometimes it's hard to know if you're actually doing that, but you can tell you've got it when both your inhalations and your exhalations take on a soft, rich, resonant, audible vibration.

To find Ocean Breath, take a long inhalation and create an audible sighing sound as you exhale through your mouth. Now close your mouth and when you exhale again, do so this time through your nose. Can you create a similar sighing sound? Practice the sighing sound in both your inhalations and exhalations, breathing through your nose, until your breath becomes long, deep, and full. Let your breath move into and out of your body like a gentle ocean wave lapping at a peaceful shore.

Be sure to pay mindful attention to the quality of your breath and how your body and mind feel during your practice. You're good to go as long as your breath is long, smooth, and resonant. But if your hear strain in your breath, if it "catches," or if your body starts to tense up, it's time to let go of Ocean Breath and return to normal breathing. You can take a couple of regular breaths and then return to practice Ocean Breath for a few more rounds.

How to Stand

Your posture, or how you hold your body in a standing position, says a lot about you, from the state of your self-esteem to the likelihood that you are suffering from lower back pain. Standing up straight, strong, and tall can make all the difference in the image you project—both outward to the world and inward to your own self-image.

There are many factors that determine your posture. Some of these are beyond your control, such as the bone structure and body shape that you inherited from your family or that were set by how you were positioned in your mother's womb. Other factors are only slightly more under your control, such as the stresses and strains of your job or daily routine at home. Other factors that affect your posture are more functional, such as the mobility of your hips, spine, and shoulders; the muscle tone of your legs, hips, abdominal wall, and back; and the way emotional stress manifests in your body.

I mentioned self-esteem before, and on that note, I'm sure you're aware of what can easily happen—especially in your upper chest and shoulders—when you experience challenging emotions such as insecurity, sadness, or grief, not to mention the mental and emotional stressors that often accompany chronic pain. It's no coincidence that your upper back and shoulders hunch forward and your upper chest caves inward during times of stress or pain. At those moments, we tend to instinctively close our hearts, both literally and figuratively, to protect ourselves. As you practice yoga, you will find physical stability that will help carry you through stress and chronic lower back pain. Because your body and mind are inextricably connected, you may also find that bringing stability into your body encourages emotional stability. From that stable place, you may find yourself better able to face the stresses and strains of everyday life—with your spine lifted and your heart open.

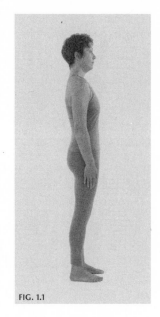

Now that you understand the importance of your baseline standing posture, it may not surprise you to learn there is a yoga pose for simply standing up straight. It is called Mountain Pose, or *Tadasana* in Sanskrit (fig. 1.1). It is one of those poses you can practice at the bus stop in the morning, in front of a mirror before bed, or waiting in line at the ATM. Standing up in an aligned, mindful way is available to you wherever you are.

Try Mountain Pose now: Stand with your feet grounded to the earth while your spine and the crown of your head elongate up toward the sky. Visualize the natural centerline of your body, from front to back, which passes through the center of your ankles, knees, hips, and shoulders. Bring your ears and the crown of your head into alignment with your shoulders. Imagine your strong, long centerline passing right through the center of your pelvic girdle; your sacrum and thoracic spine curve gently backward from it, your lumbar and cervical spines curve inward to meet it, and the base of your skull is centered on it.

Take a moment to look at yourself from the side in a mirror and see if you can find this alignment. Are your hips balanced over your legs, or do they sway forward or backward? Are your shoulders aligned over your hips, or are they rounded forward or thrown back? Are your ears set squarely over your shoulders?

Practice Mountain Pose again, this time with your back body against a wall. Place your hips and your shoulders snugly on the wall—roll your shoulders back until your shoulder blades rest as much as possible against the wall. Notice what happened in your lower back when you took your shoulders back—did it keep a long, gentle curve, or did it overarch forward and throw your abdomen away from the wall?

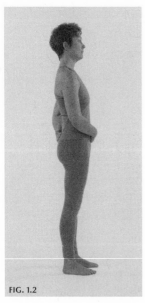

FIG. 1.2

Finally, take the back of your head to the wall to bring your shoulders, ears, and crown of head into alignment with your spine. Be sure that your chin is parallel to the floor so the back of your neck stays long.

You are now in your natural alignment. Does your body feel different from how it normally does when you "stand up straight?" This may be a very different experience of what it means to stand in postural alignment, even when you practiced Mountain Pose just a moment ago, without the support of a wall.

In your supported Mountain Pose, close your eyes for a moment and feel stability in your legs and hips. Visualize the long, gentle curves of your lower back, middle back, upper back, and neck as they rise out of your sacrum and climb up to the base of your skull, like strong, limber vines that support your rib cage, shoulder girdle, and head. Take a big, deep breath into your broad and open heart!

Now step away from the wall and see if you can maintain the alignment you just discovered and create "neutral hip position," which establishes an upright and balanced position of your pelvic girdle and centers your hips over your thighs (fig. 1.2). We'll come back to this position many times throughout the book—you can experience it by creating the following actions in your pelvis and legs:

- First draw your tailbone down the wall, then scoop it in and up.
- Roll your upper thighs slightly inward.
- Press your front thighs back toward the wall.
- Lift your frontal hip bones up toward your waist.
- Hug your abdominal wall toward your spine.

You'll see many references to neutral hip position throughout the book, because it creates stability in your hips, alignment in your sacrum and lumbar, and a healthy base from which your spine can come into its gently curved profile.

Relish your neutral hips and aligned spine for a moment. Carry the feeling with you throughout your day, and remember: when your spine is in alignment, it is strong and flexible, and your body—especially your lower back—will move with ease and grace. Repeat Mountain Pose at a wall whenever you feel slouchy, collapsed, or when you have the blues from chronic pain, as a reminder of what your body can and will feel like when it's in its natural alignment. Use it as a reminder, as well, of what it can feel like to align all the aspects of yourself: your body, your breath, your mind, your emotions, and your deepest, most essential core.

SELF-ASSESSMENTS: ARE YOUR HIPS ALIGNED?

Your hips move back and forth and up and down with every step you take. In addition, your hip bones rotate up and back, and forward and down. Your pelvic girdle is vulnerable to the stresses and strains that come with all of their movements, especially when the myofascia around them is imbalanced, tight, or weak. The result is that your hip bones and sacral joints reform into imbalanced positions. Imbalanced alignment isn't always a direct cause of lower back pain, although it sometimes is, but it can cause your lower back to become vulnerable to injury, which then produces back pain.[25]

Now that you've established the natural alignment of your body in Mountain Pose, you can do three simple tests to determine if your hip bones are aligned, or whether one is higher or lower, or rotated up or down. And you'll explore the effect of imbalanced sacral joints on your hip bones. You'll use your findings in chapters 2 and 3 to help realign and balance your hips and sacral joints.

First, you'll find your ASIS, or the anterior superior iliac spine (fig 1.3). This comprises the prominent knobby points on the front of your hip bones. Stand in Mountain Pose in front of a mirror with your fingers on your front hip bones. Bend your knees and come into a forward bend position. Massage the front of your hips with your fingers until you find the ASIS points, which are right above the crease of your front groins, and place your index and middle fingers on them. Now slowly stand up, straighten your legs, and look at your hips in the mirror. Are your fingers, and thus your hip bones, even with each other, or is one side higher than the other? Now check for rotation—is one hip bone closer to the mirror than the other?

Next, you'll investigate whether your PSIS, or posterior superior iliac spine, is balanced (fig. 1.4). These are the prominent points on the back of your hip bones. You'll need mirrors, placed so you can see the reflection of your back body, or a friend to look at your back. Stand in Mountain Pose and place your thumbs on the back of your hips. Massage the area until you find the prominent bony lines of the PSIS—sometimes they are dimpled, other times they protrude—on either side of your sacral bone. These are

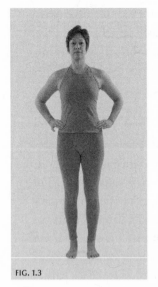

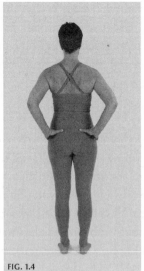

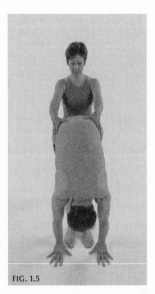

FIG. 1.3 FIG. 1.4 FIG. 1.5

usually harder to find that your ASIS points, and it helps to move your trunk around so your thumbs can dig in until you feel bone rather than soft tissue. Once you've found them, your friend can assess whether they are balanced or imbalanced.

Finally, a trusted friend can help you with the "Race Car Test," a method that is taught by yoga therapeutics expert Doug Keller.[26] Have your friend stand behind you with her thumbs on your PSIS points. Come into a standing forward bend (fig. 1.5).

If one of your helper's thumbs goes faster and farther toward your waist than the other, like a race car driver who pulls ahead of the pack, the sacral joint on that side of you may be tighter and stuck, which "pulls" your PSIS forward.

The causes—and often the results—of hip bone height and rotation difference are many, including ankle pronation, weak leg musculature, leg length difference, scoliosis, muscular asymmetry, and hyperextension or inward collapse of the knee.[27] But fear not—you'll explore yoga poses to help reestablish balance in your hip bones and sacral joints in chapters 2 and 3.

How to Sit

Now that you've experienced your natural alignment in a standing position, you'll discover how to create it as you sit as well. Sitting in a way that

YOGA FOR A HEALTHY LOWER BACK

supports lower back health isn't at all simple, and when you consider the fact that back pain is one of the most common work-related injuries and is often caused by ordinary work activities such as sitting in an office chair, it's clear that many people do not know how to sit in a way that helps their lower backs meet the demands of their workday.[28]

Let's start with a quick self-evaluation exercise. Place a chair sideways to a mirror, sit in the chair with your feet flat on the floor (or on a yoga block if they don't reach), and look at your profile in the mirror. Before you make any adjustments, observe how you habitually sit. Does your lower back collapse backward, or does it overarch forward? Does your shoulder girdle sit squarely on top of your pelvic girdle, or does it shift forward or back? Are your ears in line with your shoulders with your chin parallel to the floor? Don't worry if you're "off" in your alignment; we'll work with each of these points to create a healthy seated position.

Place one hand on the front of your hips and the other on your back hips. Drop your tailbone downward while you draw your navel slightly toward your spine. If these actions sound familiar, it's because you practiced them to find neutral hip position, which is exactly what you've just done in your seated position. You should feel your lower back elongate while your abdominal wall becomes engaged and ready to help support your lower back.

Roll your shoulders back so your collarbones broaden, then draw your shoulder blades down toward your waist, without overarching your lower back. Your shoulders should drop away from your ears—this should be a good feeling of length in your neck. Draw your shoulder blades gently toward each other and press them gently forward, imagining them as "helping hands" that support your chest and help it to open and broaden. Look at your profile once again to be sure your shoulder girdle is aligned over your hips.

Finally, draw your ears back, in line with your shoulders, to align your head over your shoulder girdle. Tuck your chin slightly, just enough to feel that your chin is parallel to the floor and the back of your neck is long. Close your eyes for a moment and feel your head effortlessly balanced on top of your spine. Visualize your spine gently curving, long, lifting, and light.

Now that you've created your natural alignment in a chair-seated position, explore it in a cross-legged floor-seated position called Sukhasana, or Easy Pose (fig. 1.6). If your thigh or hip muscles are tight, sitting on the floor may feel very different from sitting in a chair—and far more challenging. But it's good to work on floor sitting because it brings flexibility into your

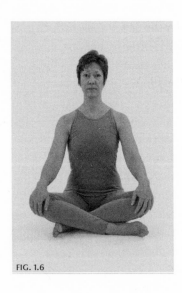

FIG. 1.6

thigh and hip myofascia, gently tones your abdominal core, and stimulates circulation in your pelvis and lower abdomen.

Sit on the floor with your legs crossed, and adjust your position with one or more of these tips:

- If your lower back rounds backward, if your knees are higher than your groins, or if you experience tension in your lower back or abdomen, sit on a folded blanket or bolster.
- If your thighs or hips feel tense, place folded blankets under your upper thighs for extra support.
- If you have knee discomfort, place yoga blocks under your knees.
- Place a looped belt around your sacrum (not your lumbar) and knees to support your lower back.
- Place your hands behind your hips and press your fingertips into the floor to help lift your trunk.

You'll explore these actions in detail in chapters 2 through 6 as you move into poses for your hips first, through your lower back, then all the way up to your middle and upper back. When you bring your body into its natural alignment, your posture—both standing and seated—becomes a tool that can help you meet the demands placed on your lower back with a minimum of stress on your muscles, ligaments, bones, and joints.

How to Rest

"First, learn to achieve the silence of the body," says B.K.S. Iyengar.[29] When I read this quote, my first question is, what is "the silence of the body," and how do I achieve it?

In the yogic tradition, bringing yourself into a state of rest is a step-by-step process. The first steps bring your body and senses into complete comfort so that the chatter your body usually sends to your brain, especially about discomfort and stress, lessens in intensity until those messages slide through you without commanding your attention.

When your body becomes quiet, a deeper and more profound experience of relaxation can begin, in which your mind comes into a state of heightened awareness and presence. A "presence mind" sees past what you normally think of as your "self"—your skin, muscles, bones, joints, internal organs; your personality; and the special, individual traits that distinguish you from others—into the layers of your inner self, your deepest self. I often think of "presence mind" as an inner explorer, a seeker of the deepest space within my being that holds my own personal truth.

When you practice the deep-relaxation exercises in this book, you won't be casually lying down to rest, you'll be practicing an actual yoga pose called Shavasana. You'll start by creating complete comfort in your physical body, especially in your lower back—each deep-relaxation exercise offers a different way to do that using a combination of yoga props and lying-down positions. When every part of your body feels supported, it relaxes and sends messages to your brain that it is comfortable and safe; your brain responds by sending back messages that allow your body to relax more deeply.

That's when deep relaxation can shift into a deep and profound experience. In the yogic traditions there are many terms that start to describe it. The Sanskrit words *shanti* (peace), *nischala* (a state of serenity), and *chitta-vishranti* (mental repose) are just a few. The last of these—chitta-vishranti—comes from focusing the mind on the flow of breath during Shavasana.[30]

Take a moment right now to experience some of the quietness that comes in deep relaxation. Lie down in a comfortable position if possible, but you can try this quick exercise sitting up as well. Close your eyes, and follow your breath for a few minutes as it naturally moves through your body. Feel how it flows in through your nose and down through your lungs to your abdomen, and then feel how it flows out from your abdomen, lungs, and nose. Visualize the soft wave of your breath gently caressing all the parts of your body, cleansing your body and clearing your mind. When you've finished, open your eyes and observe the feelings in your body and mind—perhaps they are now calmer and quieter, and have brought you into a state of peace, serenity, and repose.

Though Shavasana is often a yoga student's favorite part of class, you should be able to see that it is quite different from taking a nap (although sometimes you just can't help but fall asleep after yoga practice . . . and if your body needs to sleep, let it!). The practice of deep relaxation rests your body, draws your sense organs inward, and quiets your mind by focusing it on your internal world rather than on the external world. There is no better way to offer yourself relief from the stresses and strains of your everyday life, to refresh yourself at the end of your work day, or to prepare for a deep, refreshing, restful night of sleep.

Shavasana is not the only way to find rest and quiet through yoga. When you're practicing yoga and need a break, or if you just have a couple of free minutes during a busy day, you can rest in Child's Pose, or Balasana. Child's Pose brings your body and your mind into an inward focus. It soothes your lower back into a gentle upward curve, creating length in the myofascia all along your spine and between each vertebra. You can refer to page 22 to find instructions for Child's Pose, as well as helpful tips for creating a comfortable and restorative position.

How to Use This Book

In these pages, I hope to offer you both the motivation and the practical resources for your holistic journey toward lower back health. To that end, I have structured the book around five areas of the back body: your hips,

HOW TO SUPPORT YOUR LOWER BACK WHILE YOU SLEEP

Your journey toward lower back wellness does not end when you close your eyes at the end of your day. How you position your body for sleep is an important way to reinforce the healthy postures you've practiced all day. Here are a few quick tips for sleep positions your lower back will thank you for:

- If you are a side sleeper, place a pillow between your knees to prevent your thigh bones from tugging your sacral joints out of balance during the night.
- If you are a back sleeper, place a pillow under your knees so that your lower back can release and relax completely.
- If you are a stomach sleeper . . . consider trying to change your sleep habits! Sleeping on your stomach can cause neck torsion, which has a painful ripple effect all the way down your spine.
- If you experience neck tension, place a rolled towel under your neck when you lie down (on your back) to sleep, or try a therapeutic neck pillow that provides support for your cervical spine.

sacrum, lumbar, abdominal core, and, finally, your middle back, upper back, and neck.

Within each chapter, you will find three introductory sections:

- **Through Western Eyes:** Here you will learn how the Western medical community sees the area of the body we're working with. You will learn about the anatomy of the area, its relationships to its neighbors in your body, and some of the possible reasons why it can hurt. You will see anatomical illustrations in this section to help you visualize the concepts I'm describing.
- **Through Eastern Eyes:** Next you will learn what Eastern medicine and philosophy has to say about that area of your body. This section will set the tone for the yogic work ahead, and you will come to understand why I have chosen the poses you will soon practice.
- **Uniting East and West:** Now you will see the Eastern and Western insights we've explored as they relate to—and often echo—each other. In this section, I will offer any final preparatory thoughts before we begin our yoga practice in earnest.

Hopefully, reading these introductory sections will have you inspired and eager to bring yoga practice to that area of your body. Our practice will take shape over three sets of poses, and it will be illustrated throughout with photographs:

- **Ask and Listen:** The first steps you will take in each chapter are "preparation for practice," meant to help you discover an open curiosity about how the specific area of your back functions (or doesn't). What is this part of your back telling you? Can you find ways to relax and calm yourself so you can hear its message?
- **Practice:** This is the main sequence of yoga poses for each chapter. In it, you will connect with, balance, tone, and strengthen the area of your body—with attention to variations of each pose that will meet you wherever your ability level is at the moment. This section will always end with a meditative deep relaxation.
- **Grow and Progress:** After you've gone through the practice a number of times—or sooner, if you are an experienced yoga student— you will be ready to keep your practice fresh and expanding with a series of additional, more challenging poses.

There are a couple of ways to approach the physical poses in these sections. One is to look closely at the photographs to see how the models demonstrate the fullness of the pose and its variations. Another, of course, is to read the text for detailed instruction on the ways—often quite subtle—that you can arrange and adjust your body so that it receives the pose's maximum benefits while protecting joints, muscles, and your lower back. You may find it helpful to do these steps in either order.

There are also meditations and reflections in the practice, chiefly in the deep relaxations at the end of each chapter's step 2. It can be difficult to read and relax at the same time, so here are a few ways you can approach those sections:

- Read the meditation aloud quietly to yourself, take a few deep breaths to process what you've read, then lie down and rest in the way the text describes, keeping your mind gently trained on the message of the meditation.
- Have a friend read the meditation aloud to you while you relax. You can return the favor the next time you practice!
- Make a recording of yourself reading the meditation aloud, and play it while you relax.

The structure I've just described is, if you will, the "spinal column" of this book. But just as your spine is the centerline of your body, surrounded by muscles, joints, ligaments, and organs, this book contains some other elements that will help you on your journey toward whole health. Read on for more on some of those elements.

How to Use Yoga Props

In 2008, *Yoga Journal* magazine commissioned a study that found that Americans spend $5.7 billion annually on yoga classes, products, and props.[31] Don't scoff at that hefty price tag! Although some of these items come with cool designs and bright colors, they're much more than mere fashion accessories. Props are an integral part of a healthy yoga practice, and having a set available to you—and knowing how to use them—will help you experience the benefits of poses that you wouldn't otherwise be able to access. Perhaps most important, yoga props protect you from going too far into a pose, giving your body a little extra help so that it doesn't have to strain itself to come into the pose.

Throughout the yoga practice sections of this book, you will see suggestions for how to use props to enhance or support your poses. For now, I'll lay out the most commonly used props (fig. 1.7), with a brief word on how you can expect to use them.

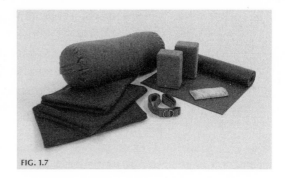

FIG. 1.7

Belt

A yoga belt, which is sometimes referred to as a "strap," is a long strip of cotton or nylon, usually two inches wide and between six and ten feet long, depending on the manufacturer. The belt usually has a cinch of some sort to allow you to form a closed loop, though many times a belt is used in its long form while you hold one end of the belt with each hand.

Belts are very helpful in seated forward bends, in which they can be wrapped around the arches of your feet to allow you to lengthen your spine without worrying about being able to reach your toes. Belts are also useful in arm stretches and chest openers, allowing you to protect your shoulder without having to struggle to reach one hand too far around, behind, or across your body.

Blanket

In yoga, blankets aren't generally used for cuddly napping (though they can certainly be used that way during deep relaxation!). Instead, blankets serve two main purposes in yoga practice.

First, blankets can be spread flat, or folded in half, across a yoga mat to offer greater support for your body against the hardness of the floor. This is particularly helpful when you are doing poses on your hands and knees, or lying on your front body.

Second, folded blankets are a wonderful way to bring height and support to your body in a number of types of poses: under your hips in seated poses; under your lower back or shoulders in lying-down poses; or under your neck during deep relaxation. You can lie down over folded blankets to open your chest, encourage a subtle backbend, or release tension in your lower back.

You don't have to have special yoga blankets for your practice, though those products are nice because they are usually both durable and uniform in thickness and texture. Having more than one blanket handy is a good idea; often I will advise you to stack blankets or roll one and fold another.

Blocks

Yoga blocks, sometimes called "yoga bricks," are used whenever your hands, feet, knees, or hips need a little extra height from something firm, not something soft like a blanket or bolster. Yoga blocks are usually made of lightweight, sturdy foam and come in an array of colors. More and more, yoga blocks are being manufactured with recycled foam. Many people prefer to use wooden or cork blocks made with renewable products from responsibly managed forests.

The blocks are rectangular in shape, which means they can be used at three different heights. I'll refer to these heights throughout the book when I call for the use of blocks, but you can always adjust your blocks to the height that works best for your body in a particular pose.

As the photograph shows, these are the three ways you can position yoga blocks (fig. 1.8):

- Low: The block's lowest position is with its longest, widest side flat on the floor.
- Medium: The next height has the block's longer edge on the floor.
- High: The highest position for a block is with its short end on the floor.

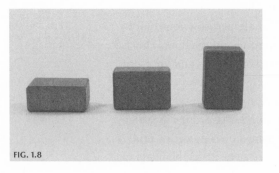

FIG. 1.8

Bolster

Yoga bolsters offer some of the same benefits as blankets—bringing height and support to your hips in seated poses, and allowing for both chest opening and back bending in lying-down poses. Many practitioners of meditation sit on round bolsters to meditate. And as you will see, bolsters also are absolutely delicious props for resting poses such as Child's Pose.

The difference between a bolster and a blanket, though, is that while a blanket is soft and adjustable, a bolster is firm, three-dimensional, and of a fixed diameter. Yoga bolsters come in a few different shapes, the most common being thick rectangles or round, log-like forms. Bolsters are usually stuffed with some sort of batting or foam, and they come in varying firmnesses, with covers that are usually made of cotton. They usually have handles on one end, which makes them easy to move around, and which can also be used as a grip during certain yoga poses.

Eye Pillow

An eye pillow is simply a soft cloth bag filled with rice, flax seeds, or even aromatherapy herbs such as lavender. It is not as important a yoga prop as the others I'm mentioning, but after a challenging, satisfying yoga practice, you will find it a great help in coming to a place of deep relaxation. As I said in "How to Rest," a comfortable body is only part of the story of deep relaxation; encouraging the mind to look inward is as key a component. Resting the eyes is central to that mindful gaze.

Draping an eye pillow over your closed eyes is a subtle but powerful gesture that encourages them to stop "looking" toward the external world and start to soften and gaze inward. A few minutes of deep breathing with an eye pillow over your eyes can be as refreshing as a short nap—or just what your body needs to calm down enough to go to sleep at night.

Mat

A yoga mat is perhaps the most iconic piece of yoga equipment. Although one can theoretically practice yoga on virtually any flat surface, including sand, grass, hardwood, or carpet, the use of a mat is advised for a number of reasons.

Yoga mats are made from such diverse materials as rubber, latex, cotton, bamboo, plastic, or a blend. Until recently, most mats were made with polyvinyl chloride (PVC), but now many eco-friendly options are available, made from naturally derived materials that do not contain potentially toxic chemicals.

Your mat gives your feet and, depending on the pose, hands something to grip so you don't slide along the floor. Some yoga mats are also handily marked to provide a measure of distance for all types of poses.

The yoga mat has metaphorical value as well, for it is the symbolic home of your yoga practice. In yoga circles, you often hear about carrying a teaching or posture "off the mat" and into your everyday life. Sometimes, after a long, hard day—or at the sleepy start of a new day—the simple act of unrolling your mat can trigger your mind to come into a quiet, focused state . . . and your body to follow.

STARTING YOUR HOME PRACTICE

Now that you have your props . . . what's next? You are ready to start practicing yoga, of course! That doesn't mean you have to quit your job to make room in your life for yoga—your home practice can take as little as fifteen or twenty minutes of free time, two or three times a week. Set realistic goals at first—as your skill and strength broadens, a desire for more time on your mat will likely follow.

Choose or create a quiet, uncluttered space in your home for your practice and stock it with the yoga props we discussed: a mat, a yoga strap, two blocks, and two or three blankets. Blankets can be folded and stacked to form a yoga bolster if you don't own one. If possible, keep your props within reach so they are accessible to you whenever you practice.

Your space doesn't have to be large—a small area can work, as long as you have space to lie down on your mat. If you like to use a wall for support, choose a space with four to five feet of clear wall space nearby.

You may choose to make your space special by having a small table or shelf to hold things that speak to your heart and help inspire you to practice—a photograph, a seashell, anything that holds meaning to you will do. You may also find that performing one or more small ritual actions, such as lighting a candle, burning incense, or playing a calming piece of music, can help you designate your practice as special time, separate from the rest of your day.

It's usually most effective to make your practice a regular part of your morning or evening routine, whichever is the calmer part of your day. You may need to get up fifteen minutes earlier or eat dinner fifteen minutes later, but the time you put into your practice will pay you back with a happy and healthy lower back—and will more than make up for any perceived inconvenience.

Finally, if it's possible, try to practice with a friend or trusted family member so you can enjoy some of the partner poses in this book. This will also help you to feel accountable to keeping your commitment to practice yoga.

A Brief Note on the Use of Sanskrit

Earlier, when we explored the meaning of *yoga*, I introduced Sanskrit as the language of ancient India. You will note Sanskrit words at a number of points in this book. But don't be intimidated! This is not a Sanskrit-based book, nor does it require any background in the language (or in yoga, for that matter) in order to release lower back pain through yoga.

Chiefly, you will find Sanskrit in the names of yoga poses, though the poses will also be named in English. Additionally, yogic concepts will be explained using both their Sanskrit terms and their English definitions, as in, for example, the case of *nadis*, or energy channels.

Whether you're feeling overwhelmed or intrigued by the idea of Sanskrit terminology, you'll be happy to know that on page 293 is a basic glossary of the terms I use in the book. Use it as much or as little as is helpful to you.

Meanwhile, if you are a language buff, and if you've heard Sanskrit names for yoga poses pronounced and were curious about their structure, here's a small cheat sheet of Sanskrit adjectives you're sure to notice again and again in the yoga practice sections of this book.

- *Adho:* Downward
- *Ardha:* Half
- *Baddha:* Joined, bound
- *Dwi Pada:* Two legs, or two feet
- *Eka Pada:* One leg, or one foot
- *Paripurna:* Full, complete
- *Parivrtta:* Revolved
- *Parsva:* To the side
- *Prasarita:* Spread, expanded, stretched out
- *Supta:* Reclining, resting
- *Upavishta:* Seated
- *Urdhva:* Upward
- *Utthita*: Extended

Here are two quick examples of how you can use this cheat sheet to decipher the Sanskrit names of yoga poses. First, if the Sanskrit name for Standing Forward Bend is *Uttanasana*, you can guess that *Ardha Uttanasana* means Half Forward Bend. Second, there are two Boat poses, named around the core word for Boat Pose, *Navasana*: Full Boat Pose is *Paripurna Navasana*, and Half Boat Pose is *Ardha Navasana*.

2

Your Hips

Your hips are many things, starting with their most general definition: the area between your pelvis and the tops of your thighs. In that region of your body, you have hip bones, hip joints, and a complex web of crisscrossed muscles and connective tissue called hip myofascia.

Hips also have emotional associations, being a source of insecurity for women who feel their bodies look "hippy," as well as a source of fear for older folks who worry that loss of balance will result in a health-sabotaging broken hip. When we want to dig in and project strong body language, we put our hands on our hips. Elvis Presley started a revolution just by swinging his. And more recently, hips returned to pop culture when the belly-dancing singer Shakira topped the charts by proclaiming, "Hips Don't Lie."

And hips can hurt—in 2006 alone there were 2.9 million physician visits for hip pain. The overwhelming majority of those visits were from patients older than sixty-one, but the second highest age group was forty-three to sixty-one, who represented 665,000 visits.[1]

You may not belong to either of those age categories (or maybe you do . . .) and you may not have pain that's specific to your hips (or maybe you do . . .). But the hips are definitely the best place to begin your healing yoga journey, a perfect entry point into your lower back. In this chapter, you will get a clear picture of how to bring movement, energy, and healing to your hips, decreasing pain and increasing flexibility. From there, we'll continue to build wellness and strength through your entire lower back.

THROUGH WESTERN EYES: THE PHYSICAL VIEW

First stop—anatomy. At their core, your hips connect the skeleton and musculature between your lower spine and thigh bones. As I explained in chapter 1, these bundles of muscles and connective tissue are called myofascia.[2] The myofascia of the hips forms the basis of support for the transfer of gravitational forces that come down through your spine and into your sacrum. Those gravitational forces move through your hips into your legs, where you literally use them to stand on your own two feet.

The bony architecture of your hips is important, to be sure, but the hip myofascia plays an even greater role in back health. Proper stretching of hip myofascia is critical to the functioning not only of the hips but also of the lower back and legs. It is through flexible fascia and toned muscles that your limbs move easily through their intended range of motion, and the nerves that emerge from your spine and travel into your lower back, hips, and legs can do so without becoming compressed or "caught" in inflexible or inflamed myofascia. You should be able to envision your nerves like tendrils of a plant that are free to move, grow, and nourish your body to help it function properly.

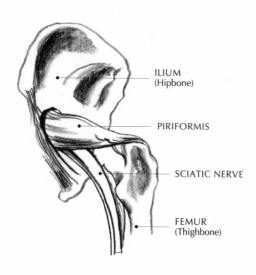

ILIUM
(Hipbone)

PIRIFORMIS

SCIATIC NERVE

FEMUR
(Thighbone)

Illustration 3. The Sciatic Nerve and the Piriformis Muscle (Rear View)

Specifically, the sciatic nerve, which runs from the lower back through each buttock, hip, and leg, is greatly affected by muscle tone. The nerve runs along the fan-shaped piriformis muscle, the major external rotator of the hip joint, so tightness, overuse, or strain in that muscle is often the culprit when patients complain of "sciatica." There's even a diagnosis specific to this condition: piriformis syndrome (illustration 3).

The tone of the iliopsoas muscle group, which is the major hip flexor, also has a direct effect on the sacrum and lower back. The psoas (pronounced "so-waz") is actually a group of three muscles, the psoas major, psoas minor, and iliacus. This muscle group starts almost midway up your back, at the base of your thoracic spine, and it stretches all along your lower back. The muscles then run through your hips along the inside face of your hip bones. They then narrow and converge to a single attachment point at the inside head of the thigh bone, or femur.

Don't worry, you won't be tested on all these details (and I'll be reinforcing what you're learning as our journey through your body continues). I'm explaining all of this here, all at once, to give you an idea of how large this muscle group is, how significantly tightness or weakness affects your spine, and how flexible and balanced hips can set these muscles up for success.

You can imagine what a powerful effect a tight psoas has on the positioning and comfort of the hips and lower back. Tightness in the psoas results in what's called an anterior pelvic tilt, which pulls the lower back forward and downward and results in an overarch of the lower spine that strains the sacral joints, which connect your sacral bone to the back of your hip bones. Weakness in the psoas can also result in a lessening of the natural spinal curves, which often flattens the curve of the lumbar spine and collapses the middle and upper thoracic spines forward. It also causes instability through the hips, and vulnerability in the sacral joints.

All of this should have you convinced that this muscle group deserves your energy and attention. When the muscles and connective tissue of the hips are strong, toned, and flexible, you will experience a confident and delightful ease of movement—imagine a soft sashaying feeling in your hips as you walk down the street, climb stairs, bend down to pick up your pet or your child, and especially when you first get out of bed in the morning. When they are tight and strained . . . well, you probably already know what that feels like.

As you prepare to begin your yoga practice, keep in mind the major muscles of the hips (illustrations 4 and 5):

- Psoas, commonly known as the "hip flexor," which connects the head of the thigh bone to the hip bones, and then to the thoracic spine.
- Piriformis, known as the "major external hip rotator," which connects the heads of the thigh bones to the sacral bone.
- Gluteus maximus, also called the "hip extender." This muscle, often referred to as the largest muscle in the human body, connects the back of the hip bone, the sacral bone, the thigh bone, and the iliotibial tract, which is a wide band of fibers that runs down the length of the outer thigh.

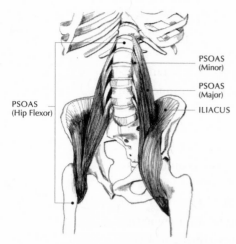

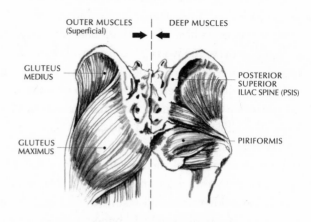

Illustration 4. The Major Muscles of the Hip
(Front View)

Illustration 5. The Major Muscles of the Hip
(Back View)

- **Gluteus medius,** a smaller muscle that also connects the back of the hip bones to the thigh bone. This is the muscle that stabilizes your pelvis when you lift your other leg off the ground.

The yoga poses in this chapter will help you stretch, strengthen, and tone the muscles responsible for the range of movement of your hips. Note—since some hip muscles are considered to be part of the abdominal core, please see chapter 5 for a helpful companion to the poses in this chapter.

THROUGH EASTERN EYES: THE ENERGETIC VIEW

Vayus: Unite Your Upper and Lower Bodies

I already mentioned that the hips are a major physical support point in your body, where the gravity that works on your upper body is transferred and distributed through your legs. This transfer of energy is deeply meaningful in the vocabulary of yoga practice, where it is called *apana vayu,* the downward, grounding energy of the lower abdomen, hips, and pelvic diaphragm.

This grounding, rooting action is the inherent nature of the energy of the sacrum and hips. It is the essential energy that connects you to the earth, and it is responsible for the elimination of waste from your body (and yes, I mean physical as well as emotional or spiritual waste!).

The best way to illustrate the importance of hips to this core concept is to trace the path of a breath through the lens of energetic movement and thus explore the yogic concept of *vayu*, the Sanskrit word for "wind" or "flow."

The yogic tradition explains the flow of energy in the body in this way: When you inhale, the energy of your chest, called *prana vayu*, expands and flows from your upper torso downward. *Prana vayu* can be translated as "the flow of subtle energy" in Sanskrit. You may recall that the word *prana* on its own refers to the universal, ever-present energy also referred to as "life force." It flows from your upper chest to your lower chest, and then down into your abdomen and hips, all the way to your pelvic floor.

As you exhale, the flow of energy reverses its course. It turns upward and rises from your pelvis into your abdomen and chest. Though we all know that our breath physically leaves our bodies through our mouth and nostrils, energetically speaking, the flow of a pranic exhalation continues to travel up to the crown of the head, where it unites with the energy of the cosmos.

As you exhale and energy flows from the hips up into the chest, the prana and apana vayus meet and unite. When your exhalation pulls some of that apana vayu energy up from your hips and abdomen, your upper and lower bodies become energetically connected at your heart center, called the *Anahata Chakra* in Sanskrit. This means that as you breathe, you can open your heart and feel all that lives within it; you can be in touch with your emotions, understand them, and express them in positive, constructive ways.

But this union is difficult when the energy of either the prana vayu or the apana vayu doesn't flow properly. In that case, the flow of energy becomes blocked or stuck, and because your energetic body feeds your physical body, that blockage can leave you feeling tired, sluggish, generally out of sorts, or downright unwell. Thus, your hips, the home of apana vayu in your body, have a critical role in your overall health.

Thinking of your hips and pelvic bowl as the container that holds the energy of your apana vayu means that caring for those parts of your body is essential, not only for your hips' well-being but for the well-being of your whole self. It's like tending to a pot of beautiful roses. In order for the roses to bloom, the container has to be wide and strong enough to support and feed the roots, lest the roots choke and wither. The roots also need to grow into soil that's treated with watchful and attentive care. If they don't, the plant becomes malnourished and depleted, failing to produce its gift of elegant and stunning blooms.

One of the most important purposes of practicing yoga postures and breath exercises is to tone and open the physical body, which helps bring about the optimum flow of energy between the upper and lower bodies. Then you create a free flow of energy throughout your body, a smooth and balanced exchange between the apana vayu and the prana vayu.

Envision yourself as the gardener of your hips and pelvis. Commit to fostering a vessel that is healthy and strong, ready to receive life force. Nurture the soil in your container, feeding it with the flow of prana, the nutrient the energetic body craves. The care you give your hips can produce seeds of wellness that will mature within your sacrum and the rest of your lower back. Let the strong roots of this energetic vine flow down through your hips and legs and ground you to the earth. Let its tendrils gently grow outward until they extend throughout your whole body. Then imagine them opening into full, beautiful blossoms of vitality and well-being in both your body and your mind.

Chakras: Your Energy Centers

I mentioned the Anahata chakra, or heart center, and its relationship to the flow of the prana and apana vayus. Now let's go deeper to examine how the chakras are another lens through which we can understand the central role of the hips in the health and wholeness of the body.

The yogic philosophical concept of chakras is that they are energy centers that dwell at specific points within your body (illustration 6). These are not physical points per se, though each occupies its own general physical region. A useful way to understand chakras is to think of them as centers of spiritual energy that distribute and balance prana, or life force, throughout your whole being. Like the physical areas in which they reside, chakras can be healthy or blocked, fluid or stiff, open or depleted.

Two of the seven main chakras are located in your hips and sacrum, where we will take the first steps on our healing journey (illustration 7).

The first chakra is the *Muladhara*, or root, chakra, which exists between the base of your spine at your tailbone and your genitalia. The energy of the Muladhara chakra is the energy that grounds you to the earth—the word *muladhara* can be translated as "foundation." The concept of "grounding to the earth" might be starting to sound familiar at this point. If so, good—that means you're understanding the theme of hips as a crucial center of health for your whole back, and in fact for your whole body.

When the Muladhara chakra is open and functioning at an optimal level, you feel secure and balanced within your body and mind; your roots are firmly connected to the earth, you feel secure that your basic needs will be met, and you feel confident in your ability to take action in your life. In yogic art renderings, this chakra is often represented by a yellow square surrounded by a vermilion-colored four-petaled lotus flower, a lovely reminder of your role as the "gardener" tending to your body.

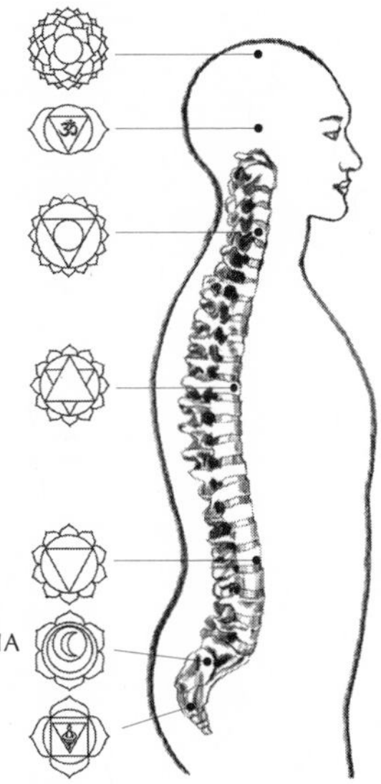

Within this chakra lies the dormant energy called *Kundalini* (Sanskrit for "coiled one"), which is thought of as a sleeping serpent, your source of transformative, fundamental spiritual power. Awakening this chakra symbolically uncoils the serpent, allowing your spiritual power to rise through the rest of your chakras and bring you to a place of deeper, higher consciousness and connection. Throughout this book, we will continue to explore the concept of your Kundalini energy as we bring health all along its path, from its root to the top of your spine.

The second chakra is the *Svadhisthana Chakra,* or sacral chakra, and it is one of the most important focal points of our work in this chapter and throughout this book. The Svadhisthana chakra resides above the root of the genitals and below the navel, somewhere in your lower pelvic area forward of your sacrum. We will explore this chakra more fully in chapter 3, but it is worth introducing now because it is such a close cousin to our current focus, the hips.

The Svadhisthana chakra is the symbolic home of water in your body, an image I love as a statement of purpose for our work together: to create physical, energetic, and emotional fluidity throughout your sacrum, hips, lower back, and by extension, your whole body. But this fluidity starts with hip

SAHASRARA
(Crown)

AJNA
(Third Eye)

VISHUDDHA
(Throat)

ANAHATA
(Heart)

MANIPURA
(Navel)

SVADHISTHANA
(Sacral)

MULADHARA
(Root)

Illustration 6. The 7 Chakras

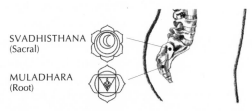

SVADHISTHANA
(Sacral)

MULADHARA
(Root)

Illustration 7. The Muladhara and Svadhisthana Chakras

health, and it cannot come without the earthiness of well-grounded hips. A strong anchor through the base of your hips provides a secure and firm point from which to take action, from which to build smooth flexibility, strength, and litheness.

With this understanding, we can view the sacral chakra as a place of open-mindedness, mental freedom, and fluid creativity. A common visual image of the sacral chakra is an ocean-blue sphere with a yellow-gold crescent moon within its center, surrounded by a red six-petaled lotus flower. The image of the moon is a metaphorical reinforcement of this chakra's association with water; it is the source of what one writer calls "emotional tides."[3]

The relationship between the Muladhara and Svadhisthana chakras is a central one in your body's journey toward health. Just as the ocean tides ebb and flow over the surface of the earth, the fluidity of Svadhisthana continually swirls through the hips and around the sacrum with the support of earthy Muladhara. The stability of Muladhara is the platform over which Svadhisthana flows, while Svadhisthana's liquidity hydrates and nurtures Muladhara. It is a perfectly paired relationship that continually balances the respective qualities of stability and fluidity. Now, through breath and yoga practice, you will create and expand the balance between the strength you need to have stable hips and sacrum, and the fluidity you need as well for ease and comfort of movement.

Bandhas: Your Energy "Locks"

Bandha means "bond" or "binding" in Sanskrit. In yoga practice, a bandha is a purposeful energetic lock in a specific part of the body that helps you hold in your body's energy, distribute it evenly, and link it all the way from the base of your hips to the crown of your head. It is not to be confused with an energy "block," which is an obstacle to flow and health. To the contrary, a yogic "lock" is a subtle yet powerful containment of energy, one that frees your body to connect fully through all its parts.

There are three major bandhas: *Mula Bandha* (Root Lock), *Uddiyana Bandha* (Abdominal Lock), and *Jalandhara Bandha* (Chin Lock). You'll learn about Abdominal Lock in chapter 5 and Chin Lock in chapter 6. Right now I'll introduce Root Lock, a powerful source of energetic support for your body in your hips near the Muladhara chakra. (Do you recognize the Sanskrit term *mula*? It means "root" in the context of both chakras and bandhas.)

Physically speaking, when you practice Mula Bandha, you create a subtle contraction of the inner musculature at the pelvic floor and lower abdomen, which anchors the pelvis and supports the lower spine. It is an excellent way to develop inner strength in your pelvis and bring your spine into alignment.

You already know that Kundalini energy exists in the Muladhara (root) chakra, and that yoga practice awakens this fundamental spiritual power. Along with conscious deep breathing, Mula Bandha, or Root Lock, is a vehicle through which Kundalini awakens. The subtle contraction in Root Lock lifts the grounding energy of the Muladhara chakra into the Svadisthana (sacral) chakra, where it mixes with the fluidity of the hips and starts to rise up the central energetic channel of the spine, called the Sushumna (more on that in chapter 3). This contributes to the process we discussed earlier, that of uniting apana vayu (the energy of the lower body) with prana vayu (the energy of the upper body).

Root Lock is a powerful way to ignite your spiritual power, opening the path for that power to flow and evenly distribute itself throughout your body. I will reference it many times throughout this chapter, so please read on to get a good foundation in how to practice it.

How to Practice Root Lock (Mula Bandha)

Sit on the floor or in a chair, whichever is more comfortable for your lower back. Place your fingertips next to your hips and gently press them down to encourage your torso to lift up. Close your eyes and draw your mind down into your pelvis. Visualize your tailbone, pubic bone, and two sit bones as a diamond shape that forms the base of your pelvic bowl. You can refer to illustration 2, on page 4, for a refresher on the locations of these bones. Energetically draw your tailbone and your pubic bone toward each other, and where those actions meet, lift up toward your navel. Draw the area just below your navel back toward your spine, as if gently tugged by a string. Visualize where these two actions meet, and lift that point up toward your chest. You should feel your hips become firm, but not gripped or hard; visualize the clear, brilliant light of your diamond reaching up like a shaft of radiant energy, illuminating your inner body.

Hold Root Lock as you exhale, then release it and observe the powerful effect it has on your body. Root Lock is a subtle inner movement, not a strong muscular contraction, and you shouldn't feel any muscular tension in your body. At first, its subtle actions take concentrated effort to produce and hold. But as your inner strength develops, holding it becomes natural and almost instinctual. Incorporate Root Lock into the poses in this book and you'll feel that it helps you carry the weight of your body. You can practice Root Lock together with Chin Lock (see page 236) to effectively stretch and align your spine from the bottom to the top.[4] After you're finished practicing Root Lock, sit for a few moments and meditate on the great source of inner strength you have just created for yourself.

Root Lock is contraindicated for such conditions as high blood pressure, vertigo, abdominal pain or inflammation, during the menstrual cycle, constipation, fever, and during late pregnancy.

Uniting East and West: The Holistic View

Let's bring together East and West, spiritual and physical, with a simple breath exercise. This pranayama practice is meant to cultivate a healthy connection between your physical body and your energetic body, and it will optimize your frame of mind to engage with the yoga poses I'll share to help you open your hips and tone their surrounding myofascia.

Start by focusing your attention on your breath. Sit comfortably on a cushion on the floor. Your lower back should be comfortable. If it is painful when you sit on the floor, try supporting your back against a wall, or sit in a chair. Rest your hands on your thighs with your palms facing upward, and with the thumbs and index fingers of each hand joined together. This is Jnana mudra, Sanskrit for "the seal of knowledge." According to certain schools of yogic philosophy, when you join your thumb and index fingers together, you unite your own individual energy with the energy of the cosmos, and you begin to understand your oneness with the cosmos and with every being within it. Close your eyes, and start to observe your inhalation and exhalation.

For a few moments, just observe the flow of your breath without trying to alter or "fix" it in any way. Where does your inhalation go? Does it move all the way down into your hips and sacrum, or does it stop somewhere around your middle or lower lungs? Does your exhalation begin at your lower abdominal area and your hips, or does it start somewhere higher up, perhaps in your middle lungs or even your throat? Are both your inhalations and exhalations full, soft, and deep? Or is one stronger than the other?

Taking the time to observe your everyday, unconscious breathing pattern is a step toward becoming a good friend to your breath, a friendship that will benefit you physically, mentally, and emotionally.

Now inhale and consciously draw your breath all the way down into your hips. Let your lower abdominal area expand—this is an especially helpful, if initially challenging, exercise for anyone who has been taught to "suck it in" at the lower abdomen. You might feel a wonderfully expansive feeling of freedom in your lower abdomen when you allow yourself to fully let go. Envision your inhalation moving around into the sides and back of your hips so that your breath reaches, touches, and nourishes your entire pelvic girdle. Visualize your pelvis as a strong yet supple bowl that receives and circulates prana to your sacrum and throughout your hips. Let your exhalation follow the reverse path, moving softly and slowly upward from your hips through your abdomen, diaphragm, and lungs.

Once you connect with the feeling of your breath moving all the way down to your hips, you can practice Dirgha Pranayama, or Three-Part Breath. The word *dirgha* means "long" in Sanskrit, which should give you a hint that this practice is all about elongating your breath, filling your body with prana as you breathe. To practice Three-Part Breath, sit comfortably and inhale into your hips and lower abdomen (part 1). Then lift your inhalation into your diaphragm (part 2), and finally lift it up into your chest (part 3). Your breath should be smooth, steady, continuous, and comfortable. Imagine a gentle, warm flow of nurturing energy moving softly and evenly through your body. Let your body gently expand to receive your inhalation. Bring your breath to a comfortable height in your chest; your eyes and brain should remain soft and free of tension. Keeping your sternum lifted and open, exhale first from your chest, then from your diaphragm, and finally from your lower abdomen and hips. Visualize your breath as a smooth, prana-filled wave that moves rhythmically up and down through your body. Practice three to six rounds of Three-Part Breath, or as many as you need to easily follow the flow of your breath through your body.

Deepen your practice by coming into Ocean Breath. As we discussed in chapter 1, this breath is called *Ujjayi*. You create this sound by very slightly and gently narrowing the space between your vocal cords. Sometimes it's hard to know if you're actually doing that, but you can tell you've got it when your inhalation and exhalation both take on a soft, rich, resonant, audible vibration.

Follow the path of Ocean Breath through your body, making the same mindful "stops" along your inhalations and exhalations that you did in your initial Three-Part Breath. Continue as long as you feel comfortable, but if your breath becomes labored or rough, or if you feel tension creeping into your body, release Ocean Breath and relax into your normal breathing pattern.

As you breathe, you might experience an energetic opening in your hips and sacrum, a sense of grounding through the base of your hips, and feelings of fullness and lightness in your torso as you allow your inhalation and exhalation to open and become present in your body. The more you practice Ocean Breath, the deeper your mind will move into a state of self-reflection and quiet.

Now you're ready to take this sense of grounded openness and proceed to our yoga postures for the hips, keeping in mind everything you've learned about how much strength and flexibility can come from bringing health and movement to these central joints, bones, and muscles.

Yoga Poses for Healthy Hips

Ask and Listen: Preparation for Practice

Before you start practicing the hip stretching and strengthening postures below, the following two exercises will help you get in touch with your hips, both physically and emotionally. The practice will help quiet and open your mind so you can begin to understand how your hips are feeling and what they might need to feel better. To start, find a quiet space where you can practice. Light a candle, play soft music, or place nearby a photo of a loved one, pet, or any symbol of something in your life that brings you happiness. Keep the yoga props I noted in chapter 1 nearby as well. Sit quietly and take a few deep breaths, mentally letting go of the rest of your day so you can keep your mind present to the feelings in your hips.

Deep Hip Meditation

Lie on your back with your hands on your lower abdomen, your knees bent, and your feet flat on the floor. If you are uncomfortable in a lying-down position, try placing a rolled towel under your lower back for support (adjust the height of the roll for the right amount of support), or place a folded towel or blanket under your hips to elongate your lower back and support your hips. Place a folded blanket under your head if you would like neck support.

Let your breath become slow, even, and rhythmic. As you inhale, feel your lower abdomen and hips expand into your hands, and as you exhale, feel your abdomen and hips softly descending to the floor. Feel how they move along with your breath, expanding upward and outward as you inhale and spreading down into the support of the earth as you exhale. Take six to ten breaths in this position.

Though we will not frequently associate our practice with specific verses from the Yoga Sutras of Patanjali, sutra 2.46, which reads in Sanskrit, "*sthira-sukham asanam*," is a good guide for this next part. In English, this sutra states, "Posture should be steady and comfortable."[5] With each breath, bring your mind inward, and ask your hips some questions with the sutra in mind: How are your hips feeling at this moment? Are they tight or flexible? Are they stable or vulnerable? Are they comfortable or in pain? Are the backs of your hips resting equally into the support of the earth, or is one hip heavier and pressing down harder than the other? What do your hips need for comfort right now?

Perhaps your hips feel "neutral." If that's the case, just let them rest in this balanced feeling. Regardless of how your hips feel, massage them by moving them gently from side to side along the floor. Roll gently from your tailbone up to your sacral joints by making a slight pelvic tilt, then release your pelvic tilt and roll from your sacral joints back down to your tailbone. These simple movements can help you balance your hips and sacrum and bring them into a more comfortable position.

Take a few more moments to check in with your hips again, seeing if you have been able to change any feelings of discomfort into comfort; perhaps you have created a sense of quiet in your hips. Listen to whatever your body is telling you now, acknowledging and honoring any and all feelings and sensations in your hips.

Pelvic Tilt

Lie in the same position as in the Deep Hip Meditation, this time with your hands on the floor next to your body. With your breath as your guide, gently start to rock your pelvis in time with your breath. On your inhalation, gently arch your lumbar spine upward toward the ceiling, and as you exhale, gently flatten your lower back into the floor as your tailbone lifts and your lower abdomen hollows and moves down toward your spine. If this is comfortable in your lower back, increase both tilts; let your lumbar region arch a little higher as you inhale, and let your hips start to lift off the floor as you exhale into a tailbone tuck. If the movement feels at all risky to your back, just concentrate on the smallest, most gentle rocking you can perform. As your hips lift on your exhalations, engage your abdominal and buttock muscles so you are supporting the movement of your hips, and lift from the tailbone first so you elongate your lumbar (fig. 2.1).

These movements start to warm up the back and abdominal muscles, bringing energy and warmth into the hips. As you inhale and arch your lumbar, remember that you are awakening the energy of the Svadhisthana chakra. As you exhale and subtly lift the base of your hips and tailbone, you are awakening the energy of the Muladhara chakra. Visualize the flow and interplay of the Muladhara and Svadhisthana chakras within your hips; the density and earthiness of Muladhara regrounding your hips and spine with each exhalation, and the smooth flow of fluid Svadhisthana moving freely through your hips with each inhalation. Visualize warm, clean, soothing energy moving through the skin, myofascia, and even the bones of your hips and sacrum.

Practice for Healthy Hips

The following poses will stretch and strengthen your hips. Since this is our first yoga sequence, I will reiterate some of what I explained in chapter 1: Practice yoga as your schedule allows. If you don't have enough time to practice all the poses in this sequence each time you do yoga, choose two or three to practice one day, alternate with a different group the next time you practice, and so on. Choose at least one stretch and one strength pose for each session. Any amount of practice is always helpful, so even if you only have time for two or three poses each day, your hips will feel the difference. At the end of your practice ses-

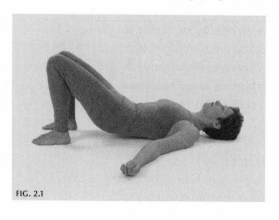

FIG. 2.1

sion, always choose one of the resting poses explained at the end of this sequence to relax with.

Cat/Cow Cycle and Big Hip Circles

Stretch | Marjaryasana | Bitilasana and Chakravakasana Variation

Come onto all fours, keeping your back neutral in Table Pose. Be sure your wrists and knees are comfortable, placing a folded blanket under your knees and a folded towel or yoga mat under the base of your wrists if there is discomfort. Make sure your wrists are under your shoulders, your knees are under your hips, and your torso is parallel to the floor.

Before you practice Big Hip Circles, you'll warm up your spinal muscles in a gentle backbend and forward bend sequence called Cat/Cow Cycle.

Cat/Cow Cycle

As you exhale, drop your tailbone toward the floor, engage your abdominal muscles, and draw your navel up toward your spine. Feel your back rounding up to the ceiling, vertebra by vertebra. Let your neck and head relax downward and draw your tailbone toward your head—this is Cat Pose (fig. 2.2).

As you inhale, lift your sit bones, collarbones, and head up toward the ceiling while you drop your lower back and navel down toward the floor. Now your spine will be in a gentle downward arch—this is Cow Pose (fig. 2.3). Repeat Cat/Cow Cycle a few times, with your breath guiding your movements. Feel each vertebra flex into a forward bend and then extend into a backbend. Visualize each vertebra moving easily and freely, with space between them and spinal fluid flowing easily through your entire spine.

Big Hip Circles

You'll come into Big Hip Circles starting in Cow Pose. Lift your sit bones and collarbones as you inhale, and as you exhale, take your hips over to the three o'clock position at your right and start to trace a clockwise circle with your hips (fig. 2.4). Continue your exhalation while you take your hips back to six o'clock and at the same time tuck your tailbone, drop your hips

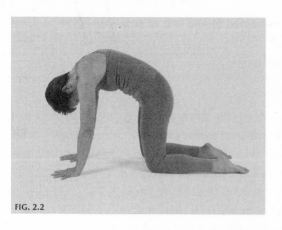

FIG. 2.2

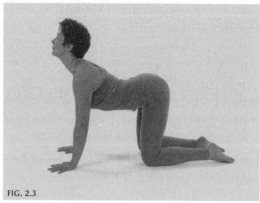

FIG. 2.3

toward your heels, and drop your head toward the floor. Your spine will now be in a rounded, Cat Pose–like arch. With an inhalation, take your hips over to nine o'clock at the left, lifting your sit bones, tailbone, collarbones, and the crown of your head back into Cow Pose, and complete your Big Hip Circle by bringing your hips back to twelve o'clock with a neutral spine. Repeat three times in a clockwise direction, then change and repeat three times in a counterclockwise direction.

This circular movement of your hips, along with the gentle flexion and extension of your spine, creates multidimensional openness within your body, which invites the prana and apana vayus to flow more easily. Since this exercise emphasizes the synchronized movement of your hips and spine, it gives your prana and apana vayus the chance to unite where your hips and spine come together, at the heart of your spine—your sacrum.

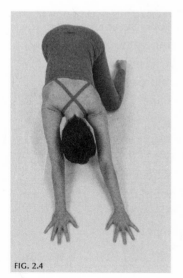

FIG. 2.4

Chair-Seated Hip Opener

Stretch | Suchirandhrasana Variation

Sit squarely on the seat of a sturdy chair with your feet flat on the floor (or on a book if your feet don't completely reach the floor) and with your hips in neutral position. You can feel when you have neutral hip position by placing one hand on your lower abdomen and the other at the back of your hips. When

YOGA FOR A HEALTHY LOWER BACK

you feel your hips vertical and upright, you have found neutral hip position.

Lift your spine up toward the ceiling. Take your hands to your lower back and feel its natural, gentle inward (concave) arch. Now lift your right leg and place your right ankle on your left knee. Lift your spine up, and then start to bend forward over your right leg. It's important to bend from your hips and to keep length in your spine during the stretch, otherwise your spine starts to round and your chest collapses—in which case your hip won't get any benefit from the pose.

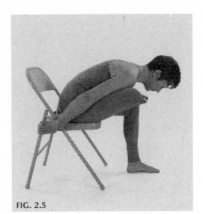

FIG. 2.5

Are you feeling a stretch in your hips? Perhaps a big one! This is a deep stretch for the piriformis, the major external rotator muscle. It releases tension and tightness that comes into the hips from inactivity and too much sitting, and it can help with sciatic pain. Bend forward as much as you'd like, moving into a position that brings a good and sustainable stretch into your hip. Breathe into your hip and visualize all its muscles expanding and releasing (fig. 2.5). Feel warmth coming into your hip as you inhale, and let your muscles soften into the warm energy. As you exhale, visualize a quiet spaciousness inside your hip, like the peace that comes to the seashore as a wave flows back into the ocean.

Stay in the pose for fifteen to twenty seconds. Then take your right foot down to the floor and repeat the pose with your left foot on your right knee.

Reclining Crossed-Legs Pose

Stretch | Supta Gomukasana

Lie on your back with your knees bent, feet flat on the floor. Support your head if you feel tension in your neck or across your upper back. Cross your right leg over your left leg, bringing your knees as close as possible to each other. On an exhalation, bring your knees up toward your chest. Let your shins swing outward, and hold your feet with your hands. If you can't hold your feet without lifting your head, support your head on a folded blanket. You will be holding your right foot with your left hand, and vice versa (fig. 2.6).

If you can't reach your feet without your groins feeling pinched or your hip muscles feeling overstretched, try a milder version instead, called Eye-of-the-Needle Pose (Suchirandhrasana). Place your right ankle on your left

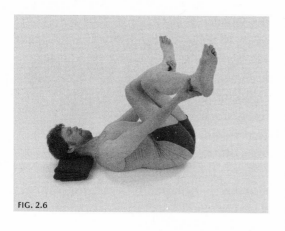

FIG. 2.6

knee and draw your left knee toward your chest. Thread your right arm between your legs and hold your left shin or the back of the thigh with both hands.

This is a deep stretch to both the piriformis and the gluteus maximus muscles. While you are in this pose, breathe deeply into both hips and as you inhale, visualize the quality of *prakasha*, or radiant light, within your whole pelvis. Visualize light, brilliance, and clarity inside your hips. With each exhalation visualize *akasha*, or infinite inner space, within your hips as well. Stay in this pose for fifteen to twenty seconds. Come out, put your feet flat on the floor and gently sway your knees from side to side. Then repeat the pose with your left leg over your right leg.

Seated Hip Hug and Twist

Stretch | Marichyasana III Variation

Sit with your legs straight on the floor. If this is difficult, sit on a folded blanket. Bend your right knee and place your right foot on the floor outside your left thigh. Place your right hand on the floor by the side of your right hip, then lean to your right and wrap your left arm around your right knee. Give your right knee a good hug.

Now slowly lift your torso up to a vertical position while you draw your right knee as far to your left as you can. In the beginning, your right hip can lift off the floor a bit. After a few breaths, use your breath as a tool to release tension in your hip, both as you inhale and as you exhale, so your hip will descend toward the floor.

Visualize your hip muscles stretching and expanding with your inhalations, and completely relaxing with your exhalations, your hip becoming a warm, liquid flow of energy that runs down to the floor and spreads around you. Stay in this position for fifteen to twenty seconds and then release the hug to your right leg, come out of the pose, and repeat to your left.

If your lower back likes to twist, deepen the stretch in your hip as you repeat the pose and add a spinal twist. Start in Seated Hip Hug with your right leg bent, and lift your spine as you inhale, from the base of your hips to the crown of your head. With your next exhalation, start to walk your right hand around the back of your body and move into a spinal twist (fig. 2.7). Whenever you take your body into a twist, it's important to lift your spine as you inhale and go deeper into the twist as you exhale. Each inhalation is a chance for you to create a feeling of "meditation in action" by keeping your body still, listening for sensations and feedback. Find the coordination of your breath and your movements by repeating this pattern for three or four breaths. Proceed mindfully, and only go as far as feels comfortable.

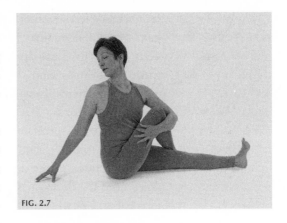

FIG. 2.7

Come out of the twist just like you went into it, slowly and mindfully. Then take your right leg straight down on the floor next to your left leg and take a few deep breaths before moving on to the opposite side.

Deep Hip Bend

Stretch | Malasana

Stand with your feet about twelve inches apart. Take a moment to stand tall, feeling your feet grounded to the earth and your body lifting up through your legs, into your hips, and all the way to the crown of your head. Bring your hands together in front of your heart in Anjali mudra, the hand posture of offering. You are now in a variation of Mountain Pose called Equal Balance Pose, or Samasthiti. Take a moment to close your eyes and come into your center, then offer this next movement to the health of your hips.

Bend your knees and come into a deep squat position (fig. 2.8). (If you can't do this, don't despair. Read

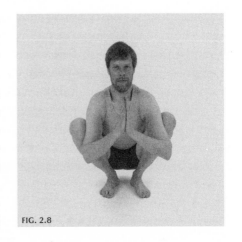

FIG. 2.8

on for modifications that will help you come into the pose.) Keeping your hands in Anjali mudra, bring your upper arms between your legs, with your upper arms pressing into your inner thighs to stretch and release them. Then press your thighs into your arms and feel that your hips are descending downward while your spine is lifting upward, creating traction in your lower back.

In this pose, space comes into the back of your hips and lower back as a result of the spinal traction you have created. Stay in the pose as long as you are comfortable. Come out by putting your hands behind you and sitting down onto the floor, or if your knees are healthy, you can fold your torso forward and slowly straighten your legs. Then roll your spine back up to Equal Balance Pose, one vertebra at a time, with your hands on your thighs to give support to your sacrum.

TIPS FOR A COMFORTABLE DEEP HIP BEND

Try one of these modifications if you experience discomfort in Deep Hip Bend.

- Stand facing a short wall that's about waist high. Your kitchen counter works quite well for this—stand in front of your sink and hook your hands onto the edge. Holding onto your support, walk your feet back two to three feet. Press your hips away from the support, taking your hips slightly back from your feet, and bring your arms and spine parallel to the floor. Look forward. Then slowly bend your knees until your thighs are at a right angle to your shins. Bring your ribs to your thighs. Pull your hips back, then drop them into a squat (fig. 2.9). The more you draw your hips away from the support and down, the more traction you will create for your sacral joints and lumbar spine. To come out of your pose, retrace your steps, slowly straightening your legs while still holding on to your support. Then walk toward it and come out of the pose.
- Here's a playful modification: you and a friend can try to come into Deep Hip Bend together. Stand facing your friend. Hold each other's forearms and walk about three feet apart. At the same time, press your hips backward as far as possible away from each other, and start folding at your hip joints into a forward bend. Your hips should be farther away

YOGA FOR A HEALTHY LOWER BACK

from your partner than your feet. Your arms should feel a stretch and your arms and spine should be parallel to the floor. Look at each other, slowly bend your knees, and take your hips down toward the floor, coming into Deep Hip Bend. Remember to hold your partner's forearms for support! Stay in this pose for as long as you both are comfortable. Then slowly straighten your legs up, lift your hips, walk toward each other, and come out of the pose.

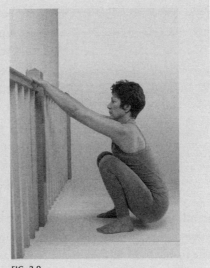

FIG. 2.9

Low Lunge Pose

Stretch | Anjaneyasana Variation

Start on your hands and knees. Bring your right foot forward and place it in between your hands. Press both feet strongly down into the earth so you can lift your hands and place them on your hips. Feel your hips facing squarely forward. This is a good time to reestablish the neutral hip position I described in Chair-Seated Hip Opener (page 46). Feel your spine lifting vertically upward from your neutral hip position.

Now place your hands on your right thigh just above your knee, creating support for your upper spine by the triangular formation of your right thigh, torso, and arms. Scoop your tailbone forward and lift up from the center of the pelvic floor into your hips. Be very aware of what your lower abdomen and lower back are doing in this or any lunge. Your lower abdomen should draw in toward your spine and up toward your chest, and you should feel that your abdominal wall becomes engaged so it helps support your spine. Scoop your tailbone forward again to lengthen your lower back; it should feel long and comfortable. With a deep inhalation, draw your

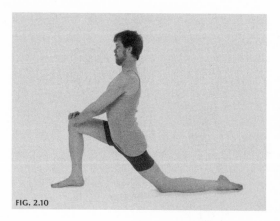

FIG. 2.10

energy up through your body to the crown of your head, and with a deep exhalation, press your hips forward and down while you maintain the length in your spine (fig. 2.10). To come out of Low Lunge Pose, bring your hands back to the floor and take your right leg back to your starting position on all fours. Rest in Child's Pose (see page 61) for a few moments before proceeding to the lunge on your left side.

Lunges help elongate the quadricep (front thigh) muscles, and the psoas, the deep, powerful hip flexor muscle we discussed earlier in this chapter. Low Lunge focuses on elongating the lower portions of the psoas, from its attachment at the inside head of the thigh bone up to the sacral joint. It also creates a mild extension of the lower back, helping it to gain mobility and flexibility.

If you feel unstable in this position, place a chair in front of you so the seat faces away from you. Place your hands either on the seat of the chair or on the backrest. Chair support helps stabilize and balance your body so you can focus on your hips, releasing further into your lunge with each breath.

Noble Warrior Pose

Stretch and Strengthen | Virabhadrasana II

Stand in Mountain Pose as you learned to do in chapter 1 (page 14, "How to Stand"). Bring your hips into neutral hip position by scooping your tailbone forward and lifting your frontal hip bones up. Draw your navel in to engage your abdominal core muscles.

Step your feet about five feet apart. Turn your left toes in slightly and turn your right leg out ninety degrees. Your right knee should face straight out to the right. Place your hands on your hips and feel your hips open and broad, your hip bones balanced with each other. Stretch your arms out to the sides as you inhale; and as you exhale, bend your right knee directly over your ankle and drop your right hip down toward the floor. As you come into the pose, keep your torso lifting straight up toward the sky and keep your arms in line with your legs (fig. 2.11).

While in the pose, bring your hands to your hips for a moment to feel their alignment. It's healthy for your left hip bone to be slightly forward of your right hip bone in this pose. But be sure your hips are still in neutral position so your lower back is long and your abdomen and front hips are lifting upward. Take a deep inhalation and feel your hips and chest broaden. Lift up all the way through your torso and spine to the crown of your head. Feel how your body stretches open in this pose, both to the sides and upward.

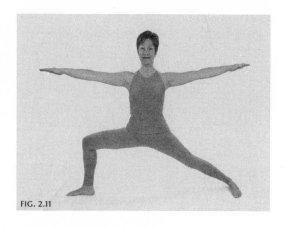

FIG. 2.11

Noble Warrior Pose is an excellent stretch for your legs and hips. In the pose, your body will become strong and vibrant, particularly through the legs and spine. You'll feel yourself becoming warm—both because the pose requires physical exertion and because it ignites the inner fire at your solar plexus that in Sanskrit is called *agni*, the fire of transformation. You have transformed yourself into a noble, peaceful warrior in your journey into lower back wellness.

Hold Noble Warrior Pose for fifteen to thirty seconds, but come out sooner if you start to feel tired or if your muscles start to shake. To come out, press your left foot down, reach your left arm out to the left, and straighten your right leg. Bring your feet to a parallel position and then practice the pose to your left.

If you have knee, hip, or spinal issues that create discomfort in the pose, practice with your back body against a kitchen counter or a high table. Support your hands on the counter to alleviate pressure on your joints. You can also practice with your back supported at a wall, which helps you to feel that your torso is lifting up and staying in Mountain Pose alignment, because you'll feel your hips and shoulders touching the wall.

Side Angle Pose

Stretch and Strengthen | Utthita Parshvakonasana

You'll get ready to come into Side Angle Pose the same way you did for Noble Warrior Pose, with your feet five feet apart, your left toes turned in slightly,

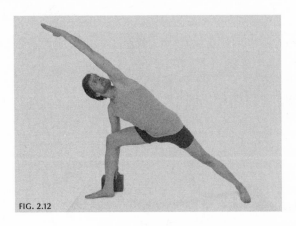

FIG. 2.12

your right leg turned ninety degrees to the right, and your hips in neutral position. Scoop your tailbone forward and lift your navel in and up to engage your abdominal wall for extra support and to lengthen your lower back.

Place a block by your outer right foot. Stretch your arms out to the sides as you inhale, and with a deep exhalation bend your right knee and drop your right hip toward the floor, while you reach your right arm and the right side of your trunk strongly to the right. When you can't reach any farther to the side, float your right hand down to the floor. If that's too much of a stretch for you, place your hand on a block (fig. 2.12). For even less stretch, place your forearm on your thigh.

Place your left hand on your left hip bone and feel where it is in relation to your right hip bone. It's natural and healthy for your left hip bone to be slightly forward of the right one, but it's important not to let it tip or collapse down toward the floor.

Now, regardless of whether you discovered a misalignment in your hips when you explored them in chapter 1 (page 17), practice a simple movement that will help you feel whether your hip bones are in a healthy position. Place your left hand on the front of your left hip bone and lift it up toward your waist—you'll feel your lower back lengthening, and you'll lift up through your abdomen. If your left hip bone typically tips forward when you stand in Mountain Pose, this action can help realign your pelvis. Be sure to engage your abdominal wall so your body will learn to hold the new position.[6]

Now complete your pose by taking your left arm up and over your left ear. Reach through your whole left side, from your heel to your fingertips, and enjoy the stretch.

Hold Side Angle Pose for fifteen to thirty seconds, but come out sooner if you start to feel tired. To come out of the pose, press your left foot down, reach your left arm first up to the ceiling and then out to the left as you straighten your right leg. Bring your feet to a parallel position and then practice the pose to your left.

Standing Swan Pose

Stretch | Utthita Eka Pada Raja Kapotasana

Stand facing a table or counter—any sturdy surface that's about hip height. With your hands on the flat surface for support, pick up your right leg, bend your right knee, and place your outer thigh and shin on the table. Your right knee should be slightly to the right of your right hip, and your right foot should point more or less toward your left thigh. If your external rotator muscles are flexible, arrange your right shin so it is parallel to your body. Your outer right thigh and hip should rest flat on the table. If you are a shorter person, find a table height on which your right leg and hip lie flat while your left foot is well grounded on the floor. If you are a taller person, place a folded blanket between the table and your right leg.

Stand tall with your fingertips on the table for a few moments (fig. 2.13). Elongate your spine upward and find your center. On an exhalation, bend forward at your hips and start to walk your hands forward along the table. You are the judge of how far to go; if your hip is getting a comfortable stretch, keep going until your torso is lying down over your thigh (fig. 2.14). You can stop anywhere along this journey if your hip is feeling too strong a stretch. Stay in a sustainable stretch, take three or four breaths, then ask your hip if it is ready to move more deeply into the pose. Hold for a few breaths, then come out of the pose by slowly walking your hands back toward your body,

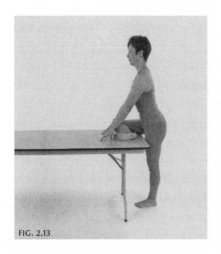

FIG. 2.13

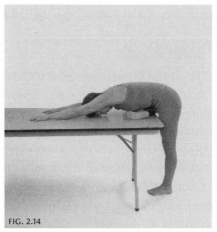

FIG. 2.14

then lifting your trunk to an upright position. Repeat the pose on the opposite side. This pose and its prone cousin, Resting Swan Pose, which we will practice later in this chapter, are especially good for stretching the piriformis muscles, helping, among other things, to relieve sciatic nerve pain.

I hope you feel a sense of openness and space around your hips after all the stretches you just completed. Before we move on to a series of strength poses, take a few moments to envision your hips "breathing." Feel how they gently open and expand as you inhale and soften and relax as you exhale. Notice your feelings and thoughts after you have helped your hips stretch and open, and see how they may be different from when we began and your hips felt contracted and strained.

A Note about Strength Poses

Now you are ready to move on to two poses that focus on strengthening your hips. When I talk about "strengthening," I mean developing tone so you can feel confident in your body's ability to carry the weight of your torso and distribute it through your hips and legs down into the earth. Be sure to go slowly at first, checking in with your hips and lower back often to make sure you are comfortable. As I often say, in yoga practice in general and especially when it comes to healing your lower back, the slow road is the best road. (Remember the phone book story I told in chapter 1?)

I suggest practicing only Bridge Pose for a week. When you feel confident that your hips and lower back are completely comfortable in Bridge, add the second pose, Reclining Single Leg Lift.

Bridge Pose

Stretch and Strengthen | Setu Bandha Sarvangasana

Bridge Pose stretches the psoas, abdominal, and front thigh muscles, it strengthens the muscles of the buttocks, lower back, and legs, and it can help with sciatic pain. It is also your "bridge" into the "Grow and Progress" section of this chapter, which focuses more on strengthening your hips.

Lie down on your back. Bend your knees and place your feet flat on the floor, about hips' distance apart and about one foot from your hips. Place your arms flat on the floor by your sides, palms facing downward. Ground your shoulders by gently pressing them down. Be sure not to pull your shoulders away from your ears, which can strain your neck. As you ground your shoulders, feel the bottom tips of your shoulder blades lifting upward and toward your front chest, an action that will help open and broaden your chest.

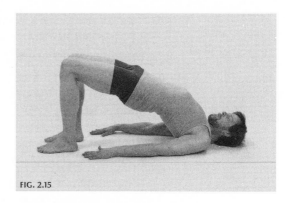

FIG. 2.15

To get ready to lift your hips into Bridge Pose, scoop your tailbone upward as you exhale, as you practiced in Pelvic Tilt (page 43). Engage your abdominal wall back toward your spine. Firm your buttock and leg muscles completely and take a breath. On your next exhalation, first lift your tailbone off the floor, then lift your hips, lower back, middle back, and upper back (fig. 2.15).

Start by coming up only as far as your lower back is comfortable. Pause halfway up, when your hips are lifted but you are not yet in a backbend, and check in with your body. If it's comfortable, proceed farther into the full pose until you've lifted your hips high and your lower, middle, and upper backs are all in a backbend.

You have created a bridge-like shape with your body, with your feet as your supports at one end and your arms and shoulders as your supports at the other. Hold the pose for fifteen to twenty seconds, breathing fully and deeply, then slowly lower your body down to the floor in the reverse order that you went up, first lowering your upper back, then middle back, lower back, hips, and finally regrounding your tailbone to the earth.

TIPS FOR A COMFORTABLE BRIDGE POSE

Sometimes it takes some work to create a comfortable feeling in Bridge. Here are three variations that are good for all bodies, and are especially helpful if your sacrum is tender and this is a difficult pose for you:

- Turn your toes inward, drop your inner thighs down toward the floor and lift your outer hips strongly upward. This creates internal rotation in your hip joints that allows your sacral joints to widen and spread, bringing space and comfort to your sacrum.
- Place a belt around the middle of your thighs. The belt should be about hips' width so that your knees are in line with your hips. Press your

thighs into the belt and lift your hips up into Bridge. This should create a unifying feeling of strength through your legs to help support your hips.

- Place a belt around the middle of your hips, as if you could imagine it holding your hips together. This usually feels good for overly flexible or weak hip muscles.
- If there is discomfort in your lower back, walk your feet farther away from your hips to allow more room for your back to extend and elongate. Move your buttocks toward the backs of your knees while you lift your back ribs up and toward your chin. Visualize creating as much length for your lower back as you can by moving the areas next to it in opposite directions.
- Practice Bridge Pose on a block to help balance your sacral joints and your hips. The block should be placed across your buttocks, right under your sacral joints. Be sure the block is not under your lower back. Choose the height position of the block that feels right for your body— where your back hip and leg muscles stay active and you feel a gentle, sustainable backbend in your lower and middle back.

It's important to rest after a backbend in order to release any tension that may have crept into your lower back. When you finish Bridge Pose, lie on your back for a few breaths, with your feet flat on the floor. Now draw your knees into your chest—if your back feels tender, pick your legs up one at a time. Hug them, move them around in small circles, and massage your lower back and sacral joints by gently rocking your hips from side to side.

Reclining Single Leg Lift

Stretch and Strengthen | Eka Pada Apanasana Variation 1

Start by lying on your back with your knees bent and feet flat on the floor. If your lower back feels vulnerable, place a folded blanket under your hips. Draw your navel down toward your spine and scoop your tailbone up while keeping your hips on the floor. Bring awareness to your abdominal core, and draw your abdominal wall toward your lower front ribs, as if you were shortening the distance between your hips and ribs. You should feel your abdominal muscles firming, which will help support your lower back during this pose. (For more instructions about how to engage your abdominal muscles, see chapter 5.)

Bring your knees into your chest. Hold your right shin or the back of your thigh with both hands, and press your thigh into your hands so your arms are straight, creating an equal action in your arms and leg. This should engage your right buttock muscles.

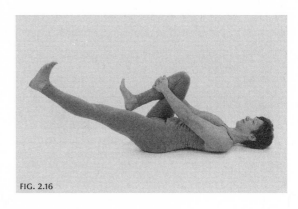

FIG. 2.16

On an exhalation, lift and stretch your left leg away from your body at about a thirty-degree angle to the floor (fig. 2.16). Hold this position as you inhale, and with an exhalation take your left foot slowly down, almost to the floor.

With your next exhalation bring your leg back up to its thirty-degree position. As you lift your left leg, visualize your thigh muscles drawing your thigh bone strongly into your hips; maintain that feeling as you take your leg down.

Repeat four or five times, switch legs, and practice the same number of times taking your right leg up and down. After you have practiced this pose for a few weeks, increase the number of repetitions on each side.

This pose helps realign the hip bone of your moving leg while it stabilizes the hip bone of your bent leg. If you found that one of your hip bones is tipped backward when you assessed your hips in chapter 1 (see page 17) practice this pose to that side every day until you experience more balance in your hips.[7]

Practicing this pose is helpful regardless of whether or not your hip bones are balanced, because it strengthens the psoas and abdominal core muscles. It brings awareness to the role of your abdominals in achieving tone and balance in your hips. If you practice it regularly, you will see a noticeable difference in the strength of your lower abdominal area. This in turn creates support for your hips and lower back, which will set you up for success in the rest of your yoga journey.

Reclining Bound Angle Pose

Rest | Supta Baddha Konasana

Ahh! Now you finally get to rest. You've worked hard both stretching and strengthening your hips, and your reward is this restorative, gently

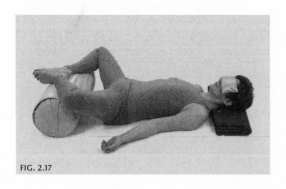

FIG. 2.17

hip-opening pose. A restorative pose is one in which your body is completely supported so no active work is required on your part. Staying in the pose for five to ten minutes gives your body time to rest deeply and allows it to open and unfold, releasing subtle stresses and tensions.

You'll need a bolster or two lengthwise folded blankets for your feet, blocks for your knees, a folded blanket or towel for your head, and an eye pillow if you would like to rest your eyes. Start by placing your folded blankets or bolster across your mat about two feet from one end of the mat. Fold the end of your mat up over the bolster (you'll be resting your feet on the bolster, and the sticky mat will help to hold your feet in place). Place your feet on the bolster with the soles of your feet together and your thighs releasing out to the sides. Rest your outer shins and knees on the bolster. If they don't rest all the way down, place folded blankets or blocks under your knees or shins for support. Support your head on another folded blanket or on a towel (fig. 2.17). If you feel an uncomfortable stretch along your inner thighs or pain in your lower back, cross your shins and rest them on your bolster.

The optimum position for your feet and legs is one in which your inner groins and lower back are completely comfortable. Before you rest in the pose, take your hands on the back of your hips and scoop the tip of your tailbone upward. This should help your lower back stay long and comfortable. Be sure your abdomen and navel are resting downward to help maintain length in your lower back. Drape the eye pillow over your eyes, if you are using one, and feel them softening inward as you relax. Briefly reach your arms over your head to elongate the sides of your torso for a good stretch, then rest your arms either draped out to the sides, or hold your elbows and rest your forearms on your forehead.

If your lower back likes backbends, you can practice this pose with a bolster or folded blanket placed under your torso instead of under your feet, and a folded blanket under your head, as shown in a pose from chapter 4, Reclining Lower Back Meditation (page 137).

Remember that a restorative pose is one in which your body is completely supported, so all you need to do now is rest! Close your eyes and let them soften deeply down toward your heart. Take long, deep breaths and feel the flow of your breath down into the deepest part of your hips, feeling your front hips opening and expanding with each breath. Visualize an unfettered flow of luminous, soft energy all through your hips. Visualize every part of your hips brightened with lightness. Feel your sacrum as the center of your hips and visualize glowing, restorative energy pouring outward from your sacrum and filling your hips.

You can stay in this pose as long as you are comfortable. I recommend staying at least five or ten minutes so you feel rested and refreshed when you are finished.

To come out, bring your hands to your thighs and manually help them to come together. Roll over onto the right side of your body and rest for a few breaths, then bring yourself up to a seated position. Mindfully coming out of the pose is as important as the care with which you moved into it; it allows you to maintain the softness and opening in your front body that you created in the pose, and it helps your mind stay quiet and passive.

Child's Pose

Rest | Balasana

When you are done with your practice, or at any point during practice when you need to rest and release, it's time to practice Child's Pose. Sit down with your hips resting on your feet and your knees about one foot apart. Fold your torso over your thighs and bend forward at your hips, taking your arms either forward along the floor or by the sides of your body. Your front ribs should rest gently along your inner front thighs (fig. 2.18).

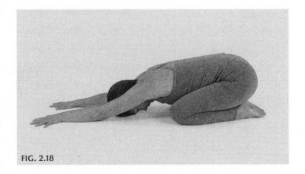

FIG. 2.18

The value of resting in a forward-bending position where the torso is supported on the thighs and your back is gently rounded is that it allows breath and life force to move more easily into your lower back. Bring your mind into your back hips and your lower back and feel the soft flow of vital energy throughout these areas. Visualize your lower back gently expanding upward with each inhalation, and letting go into relaxation with each exhalation. You are massaging the myofascia in your hips with your breath flow, as well as all the nerves that come out from the sacral and lumbar spines. Don't visualize the flow of energy through your nerves as a strong "power surge," but see it as a smooth and gentle pulse of electrical power that softly powers your body. Take the time to finish in Child's Pose after every yoga practice, and before long you will discover the restful, soothing qualities it can create.

TIPS FOR A COMFORTABLE CHILD'S POSE

Child's Pose sometimes sounds more comfortable than it feels, so here are some tips to help you receive a restful, restorative experience:

- If your ankles complain when you sit down on your feet, place small rolled towels or folded washcloths between your ankles and the floor.
- If your knees bother you, place folded blankets between your calves and thighs.
- If your head doesn't reach the floor, or if your hips can't stay resting on your heels while your head is on the floor, support your head on a block or on folded blankets.
- For extra comfort, place a stack of folded blankets or a bolster lengthwise under your torso, from your lower abdomen up to your head. Be sure the bolster is not under your hips so that they can descend as much as possible. Your abdomen, chest, and head should rest on the bolster. Rest your head by turning it to one side, then turn it to the opposite side and rest it for an equal amount of time (fig. 2.19).

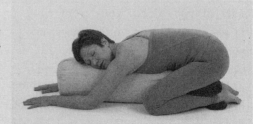

FIG. 2.19

Deep Relaxation: Move into Your Center

Rest | Shavasana Variation 1

This deep relaxation is designed for maximum comfort in your hips. I suggest a few extra props for complete relaxation throughout your entire body. You'll need one bolster or two folded and stacked blankets, two blocks, a folded blanket or towel for your head, and an eye pillow if you'd like the added benefit of resting your eyes.

Place your bolster or folded blankets crosswise on your mat, and place two blocks at the foot of your mat. Sit with your hips on the floor and take your thighs over the bolster. Adjust your bolster so your knees are supported. Place your feet on the blocks, about hips' distance apart. Check that your knees are resting on the bolster slightly higher than your heels so that the backs of your knees are completely comfortable. Your hips will be in a slight pelvic tilt, just enough so you feel your entire back hips resting and spreading outward. Lie down and check that your body is comfortable. Place your hands on your lower abdomen and feel it descending and resting into the space you have just created at the back of your hips.

Place a rolled and folded blanket under your neck and head. Adjust the height of the roll so your neck rests down into it and the back of your head is slightly higher than your neck. Tuck your chin slightly, symbolically descending your mind down to your heart. If you are using an eye pillow, place it gently and evenly across your eyes and then take your arms out to the sides, resting your hands palms-up on the floor. Finally, roll your shoulders down to the floor so you feel an opening across your middle and upper chest. Let your whole torso relax (fig. 2.20).

With your eyes closed, observe your body. Feel all the parts of your body balanced around your center. Your feet, legs, arms, and hands should all be equidistant from your centerline. The right and left sides of your body should be resting evenly into the earth. Let go of all muscular effort and holding, from the tips of your toes and throughout your feet, ankles, shins, calves, and thighs. Your inner

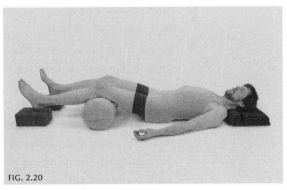

FIG. 2.20

upper thighs and front groins should feel deeply relaxed. Breathe softly and gently into the backs of your hips and feel them melting away from each other; let your buttocks and deep hip muscles surrender to the ever-present support of the earth. Imagine your spinal muscles soft and supple, rippling softly along the earth like gentle ocean waves lapping on the shore.

When you feel that your physical body has relaxed, visualize a door to your inner self opening and your mind drawing into your center. This "center" has numerous names in yoga philosophy. Some of its names are the Anahata chakra (the heart center); the *Hridaya pundarika*, or "lotus of the heart";[8] and the *Hrid akasha*, the "radiant space of the heart."[9] Visualize the lotus of your heart, a beautiful bud that faces downward, waiting for light and nourishment to bring it into bloom. Reflect on the work you did in your hips, and let that warm strength drift upward into your heart center. Continue to meditate on the qualities that live in your heart, and sense the lotus bud turning upward and opening into a radiant bloom.

Stay in Deep Relaxation for between five and fifteen minutes, or as long as you are comfortable. When it is time for you to come out, let your breath softly reawaken your body and mind. Breathe from your center outward, feeling the quiet, balanced feeling of your center moving into every part of your body as you inhale. Gently start to move your body as you exhale, beginning with your toes and fingers and slowly bringing movement to your arms and legs. When you are ready to come up, draw each knee into your chest and slowly turn over onto the right side of your body. Rest there for a moment, then use your left hand to press yourself up to a seated position.

Bring your hands together in Anjali mudra, the hand posture of offering, and close your eyes for a few moments. Offer your practice to the health and well-being of your hips, and to the well-being of your life. You can finish by softly saying "*Namaste,*" the Sanskrit word that is translated as, "I bow to you," and is often said with the intention of honoring and respecting another person's deepest self and innermost light with your own.

Grow and Progress

After you have practiced and become comfortable with the poses in step 2, you are ready to move on to poses that will give a deeper stretch to and build more strength in your hips.

First, a word of caution: These stronger poses should be approached slowly and carefully. If you feel any strain or discomfort in your hips or lower back, immediately (but gently!) come out of the pose and rest in Child's Pose or another position that is calming to you. Then, return to the "easier" poses I've already described. Over time your body will change, and the more challenging poses will be within your reach.

A yoga practitioner should approach asana practice as outlined by part of verse 2.30 of Patanjali's Yoga Sutras: with consideration for all living things through the practice of ahimsa, or nonviolence.[10] Ahimsa not only applies to our thoughts and actions toward others, it also applies to how we treat our own bodies. Plainly put in Western terms, I urge you to practice the following poses with a slightly modified version of a well-known saying in mind: "No pain, no gain . . . is insane." Listen to your body!

Awaken Your Inner Hips: Root Lock

Mula Bandha

A great way to warm up your body before you learn the poses that follow is to review and practice Mula Bandha (Root Lock), which you learned on page 39. You'll find that Root Lock's anchoring and lifting actions in your pelvic floor and lower abdomen create physical support to help protect your lower back, and the practice also gives you energetic support to free the flow of prana throughout your body.

Reclining Hip Twist

Stretch | Supta Padangusthasana III Variation

Lie on your back. Take a moment to feel the alignment of your body. Feel the centers of your forehead, nose, navel, and pelvic floor all aligned. Feel your legs and arms elongating equally away from your centerline. Bringing yourself into your natural alignment before starting a pose ensures that your body is organized around its center, and your mind may respond to that organization by becoming focused and calm.

With an exhalation, bend your right knee and place your foot on the floor. Lift your hips, shift them a few inches to the right, and place them back down on the floor. Bring your right knee into your chest and hold it with both hands. Take a few breaths here and feel your right hip and your lower back releasing with each exhalation. Move your knee gently around in circles, first clockwise and then counterclockwise, to help loosen your hip and groin. Then hold your knee with your left hand and reach your right arm out to the right.

With your next exhalation, draw your right knee over to the left. Roll onto your outer left hip as much as possible while maintaining comfort in your right shoulder. Exhaling, turn your torso to your right to release your right shoulder down any amount possible, and deepen the twist by taking your right knee farther toward the floor. Repeat this step for two or three breaths, balancing the actions so that your leg and torso turn equally around your centerline (fig. 2.21).

In the beginning, your right knee does not need to release all the way to the floor by your left hip. If it doesn't, support it on a block to ease tension along your outer thigh or your sacral joint. Your right shoulder does not need to be completely grounded either, but it should be comfortably descending toward the floor. If it isn't, experiment with taking your right arm on the floor over your head—this can be comfortable for the shoulder and give you a nice stretch all along your right side. You should feel a stretch all through your outer right hip and thigh as the twisting action of your trunk elongates the muscles of the back and releases tightness in the lower back.

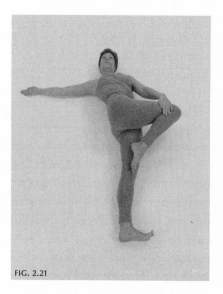

FIG. 2.21

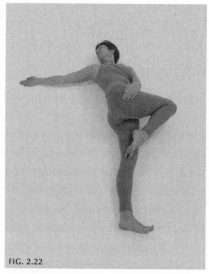

FIG. 2.22

YOGA FOR A HEALTHY LOWER BACK

The challenge in this pose is to keep from distorting the alignment of your sacral joints. To keep your sacral joints in a stable position, it is best if your right outer hip faces up toward the ceiling so your sacral joints are perpendicular to the floor, rather than leaning at an angle. As much as is comfortable, draw your outer right hip away from your waist and toward your left foot so that your hips stay in balance with each other and you create length between your right hip and ribs.

If you are comfortable in this pose, go farther into the twist (fig. 2.22). Keeping your right leg over to the left, take your left hand onto your outer right hip and, as you exhale, move your right hip farther to the left. This variation should be done very slowly, as it intensifies the elongation of the lower back muscles and gives a deep stretch to the hips and spine. Hold the pose for fifteen to twenty seconds, then slowly bring your right knee back to starting position and rest on your back. Bring your left knee into your chest and hold both knees, curling yourself up into a small ball to massage your lower back. Hold for two or three breaths. Then take your right leg down onto the floor and repeat the pose to the left.

Seated Bound Angle Pose

Stretch | Baddha Konasana

Place a bolster or a folded blanket across your mat. Have a yoga strap nearby. Sit squarely on your bolster, bend your knees, take them out to the sides, and bring the soles of your feet together near your sit bones. Does this feel familiar? Your legs are in the same position as they were in the restorative Reclining Bound Angle Pose we practiced on page 59. Adjust the height of your hips so that your knees are level with your groins. The alignment of your hips and knees is important in order to bring your hips and spine into an upright position and to help your thighs elongate.

If your hips are tight and your knees are higher than your groins, use your belt to give your lower back some extra support. Create a large loop with your belt. Take it over your head and down to your hips. Then place the belt around your thighs and shins, and loop it under your feet. Arrange the belt so the buckle isn't under your feet, and so you can tighten it easily by drawing the loose end toward your body. Adjust the length of your belt so you can feel it supporting your hips, but not so that it overarches your lower back.

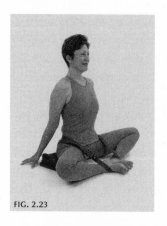

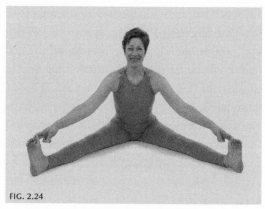

FIG. 2.23 FIG. 2.24

Check in with your lower back to make sure it is comfortable. If it feels at all vulnerable, come into the pose with your back supported by a wall. Place a folded towel or blanket at your lower back for extra support and comfort against the wall.

Now check in with your inner thighs. Are they enjoying a comfortable stretch without feeling strained? If you're using a belt around your hips and legs, adjust the amount of stretch in your thighs by adjusting its length. If you loosen your belt, your feet will move away from your hips and your thighs will stretch less, and vice versa. After you have adjusted your belt for the perfect stretch in your thighs, place folded blankets or blocks under your thighs to quiet any sensations that arise as your body opens.

Place your hands behind you on your support. Bend your elbows slightly and draw them in toward your side ribs, then slowly restraighten them. As you do this, feel your side and front ribs opening forward and lifting up. This action broadens your chest and opens your heart area. Wait here a few moments, breathing deeply into your heart and feeling it expand and open. Draw your shoulder blades down your back and press the tips of the blades forward, visualizing them as hands that offer support to your upper torso (fig. 2.23).

Visualize your hips and legs like broad lines of energy that expand outward from the center of your hips like the petals of a flower. Remember the image of your hips as a garden, yours to nourish and tend? As you sit quietly in this pose, enjoy your body, in its flower shape, as the reward of a beautiful bloom that opens up from the heart of your spine and radiates outward, offering its beauty, softness, and vitality back to your hips, lower back, and, in fact, your life.

Note: If you have a knee or sacral condition that's irritated by Bound

Angle Pose, try sitting upright with your legs straight and spread about four feet apart from each other (fig. 2.24). This is called Wide-Legged Seated Pose, and it offers a similar stretch to the hip and inner thigh muscles but with less pressure on the knees and less compression of the sacral joints.

Triangle Pose

Stretch and Strengthen | Utthita Trikonasana

Start in Mountain Pose and then step your feet four to five feet apart. Turn your left toes in slightly and your right leg out to ninety degrees. Your right knee should face straight over your right foot. Place your hands on your hips and feel your hips open and broaden. Press your feet down into the floor and lift strongly up through both your legs and trunk so that your body is stable and engaged.

Stretch your arms out to the sides as you inhale, and as you exhale, press your hips to your left and reach your right arm and trunk over to your right. This is a strong reach, so you should feel the right side of your trunk lengthening away from your hips. Now place your right hand on your right shin (fig. 2.25).

If your body is flexible, place your hand on a block at the outside of your right foot or on the floor; but if your inner thigh is feeling an intense stretch, support your hand on a chair. Lift your left arm up toward the sky. You have created a triangle shape in your body, with your feet as the base and your left hand as the apex.

Revisit your hips and adjust them if you need to, bringing them once again into neutral hip position, although just like in Noble Warrior Pose (page 52), it's okay for your left hip to be slightly forward of your right hip. Your tailbone should reach down toward your left foot and your lower abdomen and frontal hip bones should lift up toward your trunk. As you inhale, elongate your trunk to the right as much as possible, and as you exhale, turn your trunk up toward the ceiling.

Hold Triangle Pose for fifteen to thirty seconds, depending on your energy level. To come out of the

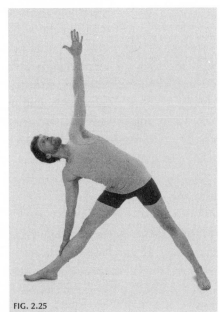

FIG. 2.25

pose, press your left foot down, lift your left arm up, and bring your trunk up to a vertical position. Bring your feet to a parallel position and then practice the pose to your left.

Triangle Pose opens and broadens your hips, elongates your spinal muscles, and strengthens your legs and spine. It's often the first standing pose presented in many yoga classes, yet it's notoriously challenging for those with sacral and hip issues. But its benefits make the pose very worthwhile to practice.

One-Legged Bridge Pose

Strengthen | Eka Pada Setu Bandha Sarvangasana

Once your lower back is comfortable in Bridge Pose (page 56), you're ready try a variation that increases the strengthening component of the pose. You'll feel more work in your back hip muscles as well as in the thigh of your grounded leg. It also helps to strengthen the psoas (hip flexor) muscle of the lifted leg. I'll offer two ways to move into the pose; try them in sequence, then decide which feels right for your body.

Variation 1: Pre-Bridge Lift

This is often a more accessible variation for most people, so I recommend starting here. Lie on your back and prepare for Bridge Pose by placing your feet on the floor about hips' width apart and one foot from your hips. Move your left foot slightly to the right and ground it firmly to the floor. On an inhalation, bend your right knee into your chest, and on an exhalation straighten it up toward the sky. With your next exhalation, lift your hips up into Bridge Pose (fig. 2.26). Stay in One-Leg Bridge for ten to twenty seconds, pressing your left foot strongly down into the floor and lifting your hips and back any amount possible. Come out by slowly lowering your hips to the floor, bend your right knee into your chest, and place your right foot down on the floor. Hug your knees into your chest and take a few breaths, then repeat on the other side, lifting your left leg.

Variation 2: Bridge Lift

Come up into Bridge Pose. On an inhalation, bend your right knee into your chest, and with your exhalation, straighten your right leg up to the ceiling. Hold One-Leg Bridge Pose for ten to twenty seconds, and come out by bringing your right leg back down toward your chest, placing your right foot on the floor (you will briefly be in traditional Bridge), and finally lowering your back body down to the floor. Be sure to take a moment to hug your knees into your chest before you repeat the posture on the opposite side. This variation can be more challenging because your hips and back are up in the air and unsupported when you raise and lower the lifted leg. The virtue of this variation is that it is highly strengthening because it asks for more muscular work, as you hold your hips and back body up for a longer time.

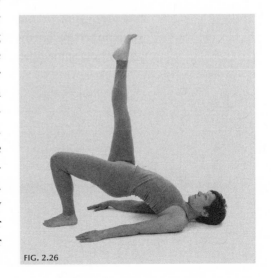

FIG. 2.26

Resting Swan Pose

Stretch | Eka Pada Raja Kapotasana Variation

Now it's finally time to let your hips release after they've accomplished such strengthening work. Resting Swan Pose—a variation on the classic hatha yoga pose called One-Legged King Pigeon—is one of the most luscious of hip stretches. With the right amount of support under your hips and a deep, flowing rhythm of breath, your hips will let go of stress and holding. You can imagine your body opening up so that you can move in toward your innermost self, like a swan softly lifting her wings before she draws herself inward and rests her head on the downy softness of her body.

Start on all fours. Bring your right foot forward and walk it over to the left, between your left hand and knee. Press your hips forward and take your right outer shin and thigh down to the floor. Adjust your right leg so your knee is slightly to the right of your right hip, and your right shin and foot point to your left thigh. Curl your left toes under, and, engaging your thigh muscles, lift up your left knee and walk your left foot back, shifting your hips back as you move. Do this two or three times, stopping for a few breaths between each step to be sure the stretch in your hip is sustainable.

With your left outer hip pressing forward, see if your right hip can descend to the floor. Draw both your thighs toward your hips—this action helps balance your sacral joints and hips, and helps loose sacral joints to feel stable. Take your left hand onto your outer left hip and press it forward again, to make sure your hips are as balanced as possible. Place your fingertips on the floor slightly forward of your torso and elongate your whole spine upward. You should feel a stretch deep in your right hip, but you should not feel discomfort or strain in your lower back. In case of discomfort, walk your hands farther away from your torso to elongate your lower back more. Slowly walk your hands forward, bend forward over your right leg and rest your head on the floor or on a block (fig. 2.27).

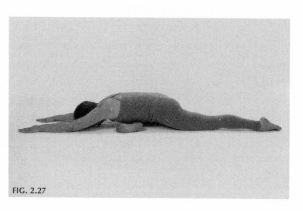

FIG. 2.27

Stay in this pose for one to three minutes before repeating with your left leg forward and right leg back.

TIP FOR A COMFORTABLE RESTING SWAN POSE

If the stretch of Resting Swan Pose is too intense in your hips, take your right hip higher with the support of one or two folded blankets, and place your hands on blocks to lift your spine fully before you fold forward. When you find the best height for your hip, the stretch will be present but not overwhelming, one that you can stay in and experience fully in your body.

Breathe deeply into your hips and feel the deep hip muscles starting to relax with each breath. It can take a while to connect with the true depth of hip musculature you're working with, so patience is a true virtue in this pose! If you have time, repeat the pose to each side and you will see and feel an immediate change—your hips should be more open and fluid, and they may drop down a little bit more toward the floor on your second round. More importantly, your mind will be softer and quieter as you rest and release.

Deep Hip Meditation, Child's Pose, and Deep Relaxation

Rest | Balasana and Shavasana Variation 1

It's important to take time to rest fully when you're done with your hips practice in order to let the work of the poses percolate into the deepest layers of your body. Lie down on your back and repeat the Deep Hip Meditation on page 42. Check in with your hips, explore them, and acknowledge the sensations that arise—you might find a very different feeling from when you practiced the meditation at the beginning of your journey into healthy hips. If there is any tenderness in your lower back or sacrum, repeat Child's Pose (page 61). Finish with five to ten minutes of Deep Relaxation (page 63).

3

Your Sacrum

SACRUM MAY BE A word you had rarely, if ever, heard before you picked up this book. That's because, in my opinion, the sacrum is the single most neglected area of the modern human body.

The typical contemporary lifestyle does not value or prioritize physical positions and movements that are healthy for the sacrum, and if you do a quick review of your own activities over the past few days or even hours, you'll likely agree. Did you flop onto the couch to watch TV during that time? You were probably overly rounding your sacral bones, "stretching" them, but not in a productive, yogic way. Ditto for all that slouchy computer time you've logged recently, which pushes your sacral joints backward so that they almost flop open (again, not in the "open" way we're going for!). Have you ever felt a broad ache spread across your tailbone during a stressful meeting or tense conversation? Those are your muscles around your sacrum clenching, tightening, and stiffening under the weight of un-coped-with stress.

In this chapter you'll find yoga sequences to make you aware of your sacrum and its role in your body. You'll discover ways to bring movement, fluidity, and space into your sacrum, regardless of whether your problem is an overextended sacrum or a tightly wound one. This chapter and the next are partners, in a way, in that the poses in this chapter may also be helpful for your lumbar spine, and the poses in chapter 4 may be helpful for your sacrum. Practice the poses in this chapter first, then move on to the poses in chapter 4 for comprehensive strengthening and toning of your entire lower back.

As you read and practice, keep in mind the most fundamental thing I can teach you about the sacrum: its root is the Latin word *sacer,* which means "holy," or "sacred." In addition to its other, religious meanings, *sacred* means "separate," and although your sacrum is connected to your hip bones and lumbar spine, as we begin to practice, I want you to think about your sacrum as an entity unto itself, worthy of your special attention, protection, and kindness. If you treat your sacrum with the reverence it deserves, you will find within it a reservoir of wellness and wholeness that will spread throughout the rest of your back and your whole body.

THROUGH WESTERN EYES: THE PHYSICAL VIEW

Your sacrum is a perhaps the most elegant example of the architecture of the human form. For one thing, it is the gateway into the central core of the body, located midway between your feet and head. If your hips are a bridge between your two legs, then your sacrum is the bridge's crown, the keystone that allows the bridge to evenly transfer weight from your head, shoulders, and trunk through your hip bones to your legs.

The design of the sacrum, structurally speaking, is brilliant: its central location and system of attachment to the upper and lower bodies creates an efficient system of distributing forces with as little impact on joints and my-ofascia as possible. Well, to be fair, that's only true if your hips, sacrum, and spine are in balance. If they aren't, the sacrum can be irksome at best, at worst a source of constant pain and discomfort that can affect your emotional outlook on life.

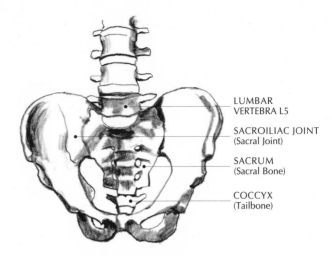

LUMBAR
VERTEBRA L5

SACROILIAC JOINT
(Sacral Joint)

SACRUM
(Sacral Bone)

COCCYX
(Tailbone)

Illustration 8. Your Sacrum and Sacral Joints

The five sacral vertebrae are separate at birth, then, starting at puberty, they become fused together to form a single triangular bone that is strong enough to carry the weight of your whole body.[1] Think of your sacral bone as the bone that anchors your spine into the back of your hips.

Each time you take a step, the weight of your torso comes down into the sacrum and is transferred into your hips by the joints between the sacral bone and your hip bones, called the sacral joints. Your weight is then channeled through your legs down to the earth. In this way, the sacrum acts as a kind of shock absorber that softens the impact of both downward, gravitational forces and the upward movement of the force of your body's contact with the ground throughout your day. Your sacrum is the very center of physical activity—and, for that matter, rest—within your body. In that way, I consider the sacrum to be the "heart" of your spine.

When you look at an image of a sacral bone from the front or back, it actually resembles a heart-shaped wedge that slides neatly between the two winglike hip bones that surround it (illustration 8). But when you look at it from the side, you begin to understand the sacrum's complexity. The top of the sacral bone moves in toward your navel and forms a concave curve as it connects with the lumbar spine. As it runs down along the hip bones, the sacral bone curves toward your back, creating room in the pelvis for the lower abdominal organs, including your reproductive organs and bladder. At the bottom of the sacrum lies the tailbone, which turns inward, toward your center, at its tip. If you trace your finger along the profile of a sacral bone, you see that it is shaped like a scoop, which is a helpful metaphor for why so many of us suffer from sacral pain when we experience stress—the "scoop" of the sacrum symbolically gathers and holds energy in your body.

Your sacral bone is hardly smooth and tidy. It's actually bumpy and curved where the remnants of the once-separate lower sacral vertebra still protrude. It has hollows and crags along its surface and where it meets your hip bones, and it has openings, called "sacral foramina," from which nerve roots emerge and travel down into your lower body.

Both the front and back surfaces of the sacral bone are covered by webs of crisscrossed ligaments that resemble something that came out of Spider-Man's wrists. These ligaments are designed to stabilize and hold your sacral joints together. They consist of thousands of fibers bundled together, connecting the sacral bone to the hip bones. The ligaments are not as fluid and stretchable as muscles—they are fibrous and strong in order to hold the joints securely together. But if your sacral joints feel tight, don't despair—these ligaments do have a little movement and give, enough to support everyday movements, including walking, sitting, bending forward and backward, and twisting. When the ligaments are in balance, those movements can be fluid and smooth.

The bottom of the sacral bone is connected to the top of the thigh bones by the piriformis muscles. If the piriformis is tight, it can tug on one side of the sacral bone or the other, creating imbalances in sacral alignment. The gluteus maximus muscles, which are the outermost, broad, thick muscles of the buttocks, also have their origin at the back of the lower part of the sacral bone and along the edge of the hip bones. Both the piriformis and the gluteus maximus muscles play major roles in sacral and hip mobility.

Your two psoas major and iliacus muscles, which run like channels of muscular support deep in the center of your body from the base of the thoracic spine to the thigh bones, broaden and widen at the sacrum like a river flowing around a spit of land. Tight psoas muscles often cause tightness and forward pull in the lumbar spine and the top of the sacrum, as well as weakness in the muscles of the back hips and abdominals.

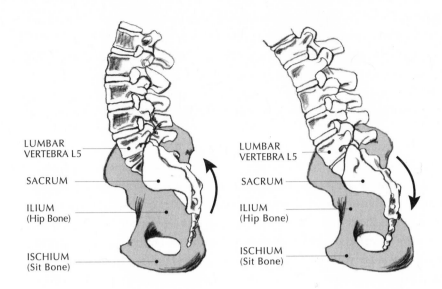

LUMBAR
VERTEBRA L5

SACRUM

ILIUM
(Hip Bone)

ISCHIUM
(Sit Bone)

LUMBAR
VERTEBRA L5

SACRUM

ILIUM
(Hip Bone)

ISCHIUM
(Sit Bone)

Illustration 9. The Sacrum in Nutation   Illustration 10. The Sacrum in Counternutation

In addition to getting pulled and shifted by imbalances in the bones, musculature, and myofascia around the sacrum, the sacral bone itself can tip forward and backward in relation to the hip bones.[2] These movements are called *nutation* and *counternutation*. If these sound like painful conditions, don't worry—they're normal within a balanced and toned lower back. But they are important to understand so you can work with them—and not overdo them—as you create healthy movements in your sacrum and lower back.

Nutation is your sacrum's way of helping your spine in its journey into a backbend. In nutation, the top of your sacral bone tips forward toward your front body relative to your hip bones (illustration 9). I think of it as your sacrum "nodding" to the flow of energy and inner power within your pelvis, similar to how I bow my head toward my heart at the beginning of a yoga practice so that my practice comes from the energy of my heart. Nutation is the natural, passive movement of your sacrum that accompanies extension (back bending) in your lower back, during which your lumbar spine also moves forward toward your front body. Your middle and upper spines follow suit, arching toward your front body as you bend backward. The result of a backbend rooted in a sacrum in nutation is evenness through your entire spine, with each vertebra equally involved. This kind of backbend both helps maintain comfort in and brings strength to your lower back's most vulnerable part. You'll review nutation and learn how to come into a healthy backbend as you practice variations of Cobra and Locust Poses on pages 104 and 106.

Counternutation is how your sacrum helps your spine in its journey into a forward bend. This is the natural tilting movement of your sacral bone slightly backward in relation to your hip bones (illustration 10). Not surprisingly, it is the opposite of how your sacral bone moves in a backbend. When your sacral bone comes into counternutation, the lumbar spine elongates and rounds slightly, and the process of bending forward is eased along the length of your spine. But just as too much nutation can cause compression in the lower back in back bending, too much counternutation can cause your sacral joints to become destabilized in forward bending. If the sacral ligaments are weak or too flexible, the sacral bone can shift out of alignment and cause great pain. You'll review counternutation and learn how to come into a healthy forward bend later in the chapter before you practice Half Forward Bend Pose and Standing Forward Bend Pose, pages 108 and 109.

Are you starting to get a picture of all that goes on around the sacrum? It's a busy place! When the sacral joints, hip bones, and spine are balanced and aligned, the area is a symphony of movement as smooth and graceful as Beethoven's Pastoral. When the body becomes imbalanced, though, through repetitive movements, injuries, structural imbalances, or general everyday stress and tension, the sacral joints can turn into a cacophony of misalignment, torsion, and tilting. These imbalances create strain and can cause discomfort across the horizontal area of the upper back hips (called the sacral band), along the sacral joints, down into the legs, and sometimes even radiating around to the front of the thigh.

Physically speaking, the goal in working with the sacrum in yoga is to facilitate its return to its naturally centered and balanced alignment in relation to the spine and hips after any movement, and to create space at the sacral joints and where the sacral spine meets the lumbar spine. This is achieved by toning the deep hip muscles, the abdominal core, and the lower back muscles. Together, these actions work to hold the hips and sacral joints in alignment.

The poses and meditations in this chapter will help you do just that; you will learn about your own sacrum, where there is comfort and discomfort in and around it, and how to help your sacral joints come back to their centered and balanced alignment in your body.

THROUGH EASTERN EYES: THE ENERGETIC VIEW

Chakras: The Luminous Energy Centers of Your Sacrum

I've talked about the amazing physical architecture of the sacrum. Now it's time to contemplate how the sacrum is also stunningly designed from an energetic point of view.

When you take a walk in a place that feels special to you, no doubt you perceive a particular quality that connects you to your inner feelings. Maybe it's the way the sun's rays float between two stands of trees and illuminate the path; maybe it's a point where soft breezes flow in different directions and surround you with nature's breath. The sacrum is this kind of special place within your body. It's a place, some yogic traditions teach, in which many different kinds of energy flow, converge, and spread out. Simply put, a healthy sacral chakra opens and illuminates the path to your inner Self.

In chapter 2, I talked about the first and second chakras, Muladhara and Svadhisthana, which are located, respectively, at the base of your hips and the lower pelvic area. Perhaps you remember that Muladhara is the earthy root chakra and Svadhisthana is the sacral chakra, which is the symbolic home of water in your body and the dwelling place of the Self. The Svadhisthana chakra is the place where fluidity and creativity reside; it's where seeds of personal growth become manifest, and one of its translations is "self-reliance." In yogic mythology, the deity Vishnu, who represents the energy of preservation within the body (and the entire universe, for that matter) resides in this chakra. He is often depicted holding a conch shell that contains the sound of ocean waves, which he offers to us as a symbol of liberation for all beings. The Svadhisthana chakra is also said to be the home of dharma,[3] which can be translated as one's nature and characteristics, or one's duty. So when the energy of your sacral chakra is balanced and flowing, you are free to become attuned to the creative energy within you that helps you find a fulfilling path in life.

The top of the sacrum is a transitional area between the fluid nature of

Svadhisthana and the heated, fiery nature of the third chakra, called the Manipura chakra. The Manipura chakra is the center of personal power and vitality in the energetic body—it is the home of heat and fire that fuels the flow of prana, or life force (illustration 11). I'll get more into the Manipura chakra in chapter 4. But it's worth noting here because its activation point is right behind the navel, and that's very often aligned with the top of your sacrum. So the energy of the Manipura chakra has an effect on the sacrum.

The word *Manipura* means "city of gems." When it is open and balanced, your Manipura chakra is a place of luminosity and energy that fuels life—it's your personal sun, contained but powerful, and it illuminates your path toward self-activation. When it's out of balance, energetically speaking, there's too much heat and fire in your body. In this holistic view, "burning" or "hot" pain in your sacrum may be your body's way of letting you know that your Manipura chakra needs some attention.

There are many reasons the Manipura chakra may be out of balance. Muscular tightness in the deep hip muscles and the lower back due to injury, musculoskeletal imbalances, or unhealthy posture may restrict its energy. Stressors in everyday life and pressures in the workplace (and the accompanying poor sitting and standing postures those things usually bring) can turn into gripping and stiffening in the sacrum.

Yet we all know that sometimes the causes of imbalances in the body are next to impossible to figure out! Luckily for us, though, the energy of the Manipura chakra flows down into the Svadhisthana chakra. Energetically speaking, the watery nature of Svadhisthana balances the fire of Manipura, and the result is a practical energy that helps to transform your ideas of self-fulfillment into reality. Next time you get a "gut feeling," imagine this balancing action between your two chakras, and visualize your sacrum as the vessel that holds them in balanced relationship with each other.

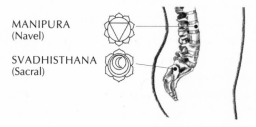

MANIPURA
(Navel)

SVADHISTHANA
(Sacral)

Illustration 11. The Svadhisthana and Manipura Chakras

Nadis: Rivers of Inner Energy

I mentioned earlier that the psoas muscles are like channels of muscular support that run the length of your middle and lower body. Yogic philosophy teaches that you also have channels, or rivers, of energy, called *nadis* in Sanskrit, which run throughout your body. The network of nadis is a complex three-dimensional web that carries prana to every part of your body. According to yogic texts, there are at least 72,000 of these rivers of energy flowing through your body.[4] The three largest nadis are called, in Sanskrit, *Ida, Pingala,* and *Sushumna,* and each is part of the energetic story of your sacrum (illustration 12).

Let's start with the Sushumna, which is considered to be the major channel of subtle energy in the body. It begins at the Muladhara (root) chakra and runs up through your spine all the way to the Sahasrara chakra at the crown of your head

In yogic mythology, you may remember from chapter 2, the source of the body's subtle energy is called Kundalini, which means "coiled one." Kundalini is often depicted in the form of a serpent-like goddess, who sleeps coiled up in her resting place in the Muladhara chakra. One of the goals of yoga practice is to awaken the power of Kundalini energy. This energy, once activated, courses through all of the chakras, and as it passes through each one, it energizes that area of the body, clearing a path for subtle energy to flow upward through the Sushumna into the crown chakra, where we ultimately realize our unity with the cosmos and experience self-realization.

The flow of Kundalini-fueled prana through a nadi like the Sushumna can be palpable to a yoga practitioner. If you've practiced yoga and felt that the poses and breathing exercises have awakened something deep inside you, leaving yoiu feeling energized, balanced, and self-reflective, you may have purified and cleansed your nadis and allowed fresh energy to flow freely through them.

When you lie down to rest in deep relaxation at the end of a yoga class, you may become aware of a cyclical flow of energy through the Sushumna. This flow starts at your sacrum, moves up your spine into your head, and then goes back down to your sacrum, repeating itself over and over. The flow is continuous, like the ever-present motion of ocean waves or a rhythmic pulse. Being aware of the flow of prana through the Sushumna is a peaceful, joyful experience. It is a feeling that all the parts of yourself have come together in a feeling of unity and are intimately and inextricably connected to the rhythms of the natural world.

The other two major nadis surround the Sushumna and complement each other. The Ida is called the "lunar" channel because it is associated with passivity, reflectivity, and cooling. It corresponds to the left side of the body and the right side of the brain. The Pingala is called the "solar" channel because it is associated with the qualities of action, movement, and heat. It corresponds to the right side of the body and the left side of the brain. Both Ida and Pingala start at the Muladhara chakra and wind their way up the Sushumna, crossing at each chakra.

Can you guess where these two nadis make their first crossing? At the sacral plexus, the Svadhisthana chakra! When they meet, Ida, Pingala, and Sushumna join and awaken the powerful energies of your sacrum that help you feel vital, alive, energized, and present. When they meet again at the Manipura chakra, behind your navel, the fiery power of your personal sun is energized, illuminating your path.

Your sacrum is an amazing convergence of physical and energetic forces in your body. Close your eyes and take a moment to visualize the weblike physical structure of the ligaments that hold your sacral joints in place, and how it is juxtaposed with the smooth, serpentine flow of subtle energy through Ida and Pingala as those nadis make their way up and around the Sushumna.

These elements are all part of your sacral "orchestra." When they are in tune with one another, there is communication and coordination among them and you feel ease and harmony in your sacrum. When the energy is blocked or imbalanced, whether physically or energetically, the members of the orchestra can't hear one another; they can't find the right rhythm for their instruments. Imbalances and blockages can manifest as feelings such as "Whose body is this, anyway, because it sure doesn't feel like mine?" at best, moving into discomfort and debilitating pain at worst. The earlier you can notice signs of disconnect in your sacrum, the better you'll be able to ensure your sacral orchestra stays smooth and melodious. With your yoga practice, you will learn how to help it to become a symphony of movement and fluidity.

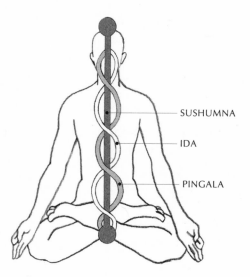

SUSHUMNA

IDA

PINGALA

Illustration 12. The Three Major *Nadis*

Uniting East and West: The Holistic View

Every sacrum is different, and given the complexity we've described so far in this chapter, you can imagine a number of ways that your sacrum can ache, pull, clench, stab, and generally bother you. Before you begin your yoga practice to create sacral balance, let's go over three of the most common issues that may be afflicting your sacrum.

This section might seem like it's simply more information about the physical body—the Western perspective—but really, I see the details below as an invitation to put East and West together and enable you to fully listen to what your sacrum is trying to tell you. Remember that, holistically speaking, your energetic body can't thrive and your nadis can't flow when your physical body is injured or compromised, and you can't help your physical body heal unless you are accurately informed and deeply connected with its specific challenges.

Sacral Sprain

When pain spreads more or less evenly across the back of your hips along the sacral band, it may be due to what is called a sacral sprain. A sacral sprain can be due to strain in the muscles around the hips or injury to the sacral ligaments. It can start as a feeling of mild discomfort or a dull ache; if not attended to, it will worsen over time. It can cause the musculature of the hips and lower back to tighten up and sometimes go into spasm. Because there are so many nerve endings in the sacrum that are sensitive to how your weight is distributed through your sacrum, even a mild sacral sprain can be quite painful. If you have a sacral sprain, sitting may be the most stressful position for your sacrum and lower back. Movement in either forward-bending or back-bending directions can seem almost impossible, while twisting and side-bending movements may be less affected.[5]

Referred or Radiating Sacral Pain

Another pain pattern due to sacral ligament injuries is when pain radiates down one side of the back hip toward the knee, or radiates through both sides of the hips. This pain can take many forms; it can be sharp and acute, or it can be a nagging, chronic, low-level achiness.

A challenge of working with referred and radiating sacral pain is that the pain patterns can be complex and more difficult to diagnose than straightforward pain across the sacral band. In one body, forward bending may exacerbate an injury, while in another body the same movement may help alleviate pain. If you have referred or radiating sacral pain, it's important to track which movements affect your pain, and how. If you listen to your body, you will be able to discern when the sensations you feel are good and healthy—the kind that help to tone and strengthen the musculature—because your body will feel better after you do those poses. Tuning in to how your body lets you move (and what it doesn't like) may help you trace the sources of your radiating and referred pain.

Sacral Joint Pain

Focused pain in one or both of your sacral joints may be due to rotation and torsion in the position of your hip or sacral bones or compression (downward force) of your sacral bone into the sacral joints. Repeating the pelvic self-assessment I explained on page 17 can help you determine whether skeletal imbalances might be the culprit in your sacral joint pain. Like sacral sprains, sacral joint imbalances can start out as minor shifts in the alignment of your hips and sacrum, and they can grow worse over time. Conversely, sometimes an extreme movement or sudden jolt to your hips pushes the joints over the edge, resulting in acute pain. More commonly, sacral joint issues are due to chronic imbalance: One sacral joint can be overstretched and the other can be compressed; one side can shift or tilt backward while the other side shifts forward.

Pain due to an imbalance in the sacral joints can feel quite different from that of a sacral sprain. It is often specific to one side or the other. Yoga poses in which the hips are externally rotated (turned outward), such as Triangle Pose or Seated Bound Angle Pose, can irritate sacral joint pain. Forward-bending or back-bending movements might feel fairly comfortable, but twisting and side-bending movements can exacerbate pain in an achy joint.

These three sacral maladies—sacral sprain, referred/radiating pain, and sacral joint pain—are not mutually exclusive. In fact, whatever the cause of your sacral discomfort is, the musculature in the general area may become imbalanced and weak, and your sacral joints can become unstable.

Your body will let you know that it needs help bringing your sacrum back into balance.

Of course, your sacral issues may not fall into any of the three categories I mentioned above. There are, however, some simple ways you can make a more educated guess on whether your sacral joints are overstretched, inflexible, or imbalanced. As you develop your personal yoga practice, you can experiment with different categories of movements to discover which poses help soothe your sacrum. Generally speaking:

- Backbends can help strengthen the muscles that support the hips and the sacral joints. They are helpful in "drawing things together" when ligaments have become overstretched or imbalanced.
- Forward bends can help release muscular tightness in the back hips and the sacral band.
- Twists lengthen the myofascia around the hips and the lower back.
- Tractioning, or drawing the spine away from the hips, helps release compression in the sacral joints.

You can see that, depending on your sacrum's condition, backbends, forward bends, or both can be particularly challenging and uncomfortable. Because they figure so prominently into the big picture of yoga, I'll focus on each so you learn how to practice them safely and comfortably while you help your sacrum heal.

Backbends and Your Sacrum

Backbends are excellent for balancing your sacral joints, strengthening the back of your hips and lower back, and lengthening your psoas major muscle, all of which are crucial for sacral health. Backbends are perfect for when your sacral joints feel pulled, twisted, or overstretched. They complement the poses that work on abdominal core strength by balancing the strength of the front and back bodies, creating muscular balance through and through.

It's important, when you are about to attempt a backbend pose, to remember that a tight muscle isn't necessarily strong; strong muscles are able to do their job of supporting your body, yet they are flexible at the same time in order to allow for a comfortable range of motion. A tight muscle, on the other hand, even though it feels taut, can be weak and vulnerable to injury. Strong yet flexible muscles are what help your spine come into an evenly curved backbend from the top of your sacral joints all the way up to the nape of the neck. Therefore, because backbends can contribute to compression in the lower back, caution is advised when the lower back musculature is tight or in spasm.

When practicing any of the backbends in this book, always come into the pose slowly, and proceed mindfully. Feel and listen to your sacrum while you move into, stay in, and come out of each pose. Initially a backbend will feel best for an overstretched rather than a tight or gripped lower back. Eventually, with time and practice, any lower back will feel good in, and benefit from, backbends.

Remember, you don't need to do an extreme backbend in order to get the benefits. In fact, if you are trying to heal a sacral injury, smaller movements feel better, and may even be more therapeutic because they reshape your musculature incrementally, a little at a time, giving your body time to adjust to and maintain its new, balanced alignment. When your sacrum gives you the "thumbs up" signal that it feels happy and comfortable, start to increase the arch in your back and move more deeply into the poses. When you practice the backbend sequence in this chapter, be sure to take breaks between poses so any tension in your lower back releases. Practice Cat/Cow Cycle (page 45) or Free-Your-Sacrum Pose (page 94).

Forward Bends and Your Sacrum

The idea of lengthening and releasing your sacral joints in a forward bend sounds delicious, but if you've ever had a tight or destabilized feeling in your sacrum, you know how challenging it can be to find comfort while bending forward. It is important to learn how to come into a forward bend properly by bending at your hip joints rather than rounding forward from your back. Forward bends should be practiced with caution when your sacral joints are overstretched and imbalanced.

A healthy forward bend will create length in the sacral joints and lumbar spine, and maintain the integrity of your sacral joints.

Try the following little experiment to feel this in your own body. Stand tall with your feet about hips' distance apart. Place your fingertips right where your thighs meet your hips, at the crease of your front groins. Without pivoting your feet, turn your upper thighs inward so your pubic bone starts to move back toward your tailbone. Start to bend forward and feel what happens in your groins and to your fingers. Do your groins soften and deepen back toward your back hips and do your fingers move deeply into the soft folds of the skin and myofascia? This is the feeling you want in a forward bend, the feeling that your hip musculature is able to soften and release, bending from the hip joints.

If you can't get this feeling and find that the forward bend is happening somewhere in your lower or middle back, your hamstring muscles may be tight. Your hamstrings are three long muscles that begin at your sit bones, run along the backs of your thighs, along the backs of your knees, and connect to your lower leg. They are what allow your knees to flex and extend.[6] But if they're tight, they can inhibit your ability to bend forward from your hips. If this happens in your body, try again, this time disengaging your hamstrings by bending your knees. Can you feel the fold at your front hip creases now? Once you're comfortable in your bend, slowly and mindfully straighten your legs one at a time and notice any changes in your body position. Were you able to keep the bend at your hips as you straightened your legs, or did the bend move up from your hips into your lower and middle back?

This should be an *aha!* moment—now you can understand the relationship between your hips and hamstrings, and their effects on your sacrum. Practicing yoga will lengthen your hamstrings and tone your hip flexors so that over time you will be able to maintain forward folding from your hip joints.

The most important thing you can do as you experience the practice in this chapter is to be kind to your sacrum. Even though I just described movements to release and strengthen your sacrum, you may find that twisting, for example, irritates your already tender sacral band. Listen to your body, and give it permission to hold off on poses that bring pain or discomfort. Remember the maxim that health is a journey as well as a destination—as you grow in your practice, you will find yourself able to do more and more movements, and to do them in more and more comfort. Your sacrum is an incredibly complex area, and it can take a bit of patient self-study to find out what will help it heal.

Long-lasting sacral wellness is a combination of balanced strength and flexibility of the myofascia, joint mobility, and structural alignment. When you create wellness in your physical sacrum, you pave the way for wellness in the energetic channels we discussed—the Ida, Pingala, and Sushumna—so that powerful Kundalini energy can flow easily through the Svadhisthana (sacral) chakra. Listening to the messages from your sacrum will help you to understand what is happening and what it needs; then you can embark on your journey to bring health to the heart of your spine.

Yoga Poses for a Healthy Sacrum

Ask and Listen: Preparation for Practice

Standing Sacral Meditation

Stand tall with your feet about hips' distance apart, and bring your body into its natural alignment. Take your hands onto the back of your hips and place your thumbs on your sacral joints. Gently massage the joints with your thumbs and observe the feelings that come, asking yourself some questions to help you discern the condition of your sacral joints. Be sure to simply observe the sensations as you do this exercise; do not let judgment or anxiety color your exploration. Sway your hips gently to one side and then to the other and contemplate these questions:

- Are your sacral joints comfortable?
- Do they feel even with each other, or does one side feel higher, lower, or farther back than the other?
- Do you feel soreness, tenderness, or pain on one side or the other?

Now take your hands so your fingers face downward on your buttocks, supporting your sacral joints in the palms of your hands. Experiment with very gentle back-bending, forward-bending, and twisting movements, and observe how your lower back feels. When you come into a slight backbend, is there pain at your sacral band, the horizontal area that goes across your sacral joints, or does the motion feel soothing? Do you even feel a bend at your sacral joints, or do they stiffen as your body instinctively goes into an arch in your lower back? How does it feel when you bend forward? How does it feel in your sacral joints when you bend to the right and to the left? When you twist to the right and to the left? If pain comes in any of these movements, don't push farther into them; the work here is to simply note what triggers your pain.

As you move your trunk around your hips, making mental notes of which actions feel comfortable and which cause discomfort, begin to visualize the specific imbalances in your sacral joints. Now as you practice poses to help with sacral pain, you can include only those that help you feel better, and let go of ones that create discomfort. As your sacrum becomes stronger and more stable, you'll be able to add those poses back into your sequence, and you will experience them with comfort.

Doorway Stand

Find an opening between two walls or a doorway that's between three and four feet wide. Stand against one side of the opening. If it is a narrow doorframe, be sure your sacral joints are both fully supported. If the doorframe isn't flat, place a sturdy book behind your hips so you can feel both hips evenly pressing into the surface you are standing against. Place your hands on your hips and bring them into neutral position, with your hips level both to the floor and against the doorway. The goal, if possible in your body, is to start this pose with your hips and sacral joints all in alignment, and with your lumbar spine in its natural, gentle inward curve.

Bend your right knee and lift your right leg up, bringing your foot against the other side of the doorway. Place your foot directly opposite your right hip, or as close as you can get while keeping your hips level and maintaining the natural curve of your lumbar spine, then press your foot into the doorframe (fig. 3.1). Mentally examine your hips. What happened when you lifted your foot? Did your hips stay level, or did your right hip hike up, shortening the musculature on the right side of your back and torso? Rebalance your hips if that's the case in your body. Now explore the feeling in your right sacral joint. Is it balanced with your left side? Is it pressing more strongly into the wall than your left joint? Is it achy or uncomfortable? Move your hips around, up and down and back and forth, and see if you can determine any imbalances in your sacral joints. Hold for about a minute and then release and repeat on your left side.

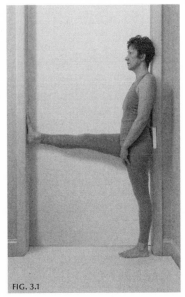

FIG. 3.1

Doorway Stand is another excellent opportunity to explore imbalances in your hips and sacral joints, and to learn how to bring them into balance. For example, say your right side is achy and uncomfortable when you practice the pose to your right, but when you practice on the left side, your left sacral joint is comfortable. This indicates that your right joint may be shifted backward and out of alignment with your hips. If this example applies to you, try to gently press your right sacral joint forward while you press your left hip back into the wall. Try both sides again and see if you can observe any change.

Sacral Circles

Lie on the floor (not on a mat) with your knees bent and your feet flat on the floor, about hips' width apart. If you are lying on a soft surface such as a plush rug, place a large, flat book under your hips. Moving from your pelvis rather than your legs, lean slightly into your right hip and trace the outline of your right sacral joint into the floor, starting from your tailbone and moving up along the joint to the top of the hip bone. Follow the circle over to your left and move down along the left sacral joint, ending back at your tailbone. Trace three circles starting on your right side. Change direction and trace three circles starting on your left side.

Explore how each side of your sacrum feels as you move it along the floor. Note if there is comfort or discomfort as each joint gets its massage. Does one side of the sacrum press more strongly into the floor than the other? If so, that joint may be rotated backward; the hip bone on that side may also be rotated back, or the opposite hip bone may be rotated forward. This exercise provides information about imbalances in the pelvis and gives a gentle therapeutic and stimulating massage to the myofascia. It's an opportunity for tight sacral joints and an overarched lower back to experience release as you roll your sacral joints and lower back flat on the floor. If you practice Sacral Circles every day, you may find that compressed sacral joints relax and become more comfortable.

Note: Sacral "circles" might actually be a misnomer for this pose, as the sacrum is actually shaped more like a heart than a circle, coming to a rounded indentation at the top, and joining together at the "point" of your very-low spine at the bottom. As you do this pose, you may wish to imagine tracing a heart with your movements, and visualize what it means to you to be delving more deeply into "the heart of your spine."

Reclining Knee Squeeze

Lie on your back with your feet flat on the floor, a little more than hips' width apart. Keeping your hips on the floor, lift your tailbone slightly up toward the ceiling. Draw your frontal hip bones up toward your ribs while your navel drops toward your spine. Feel your abdominal core muscles engaging. Your lumbar spine will gently press along the floor.

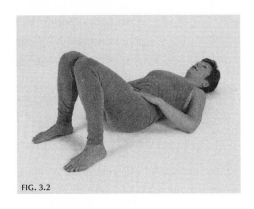

FIG. 3.2

Press your knees together for fifteen to twenty seconds, then release the action and observe the feeling across your sacrum (fig. 3.2). The action of pressing your knees together releases your piriformis muscles and helps to release tightness and compression in your sacral joints. Reclining Knee Squeeze gives a feeling of openness along the sacral band. It feels good if your sacrum is tight or compressed and it may also help sciatic pain. Repeat three to four times, each time observing any amount of release in your sacral band.

Practice for a Healthy Sacrum

Happy Baby Pose

Stretch | Dwi Pada Apanasana Variation 1

Lie on your back and bring your knees toward your chest. Opening your knees out to the sides, near your armpits, bring your hands inside your legs and hold your big toes. Keeping your knees near your side chest and armpits, lift your shins up so the soles of your feet are parallel to the ceiling (fig. 3.3). If you can't come into this position maintaining the hold of your big toes, wrap belts around your feet instead.

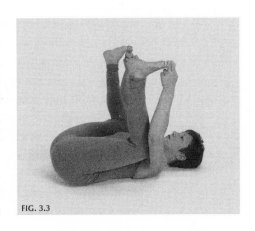

FIG. 3.3

Take five or six big deep breaths, and with each exhalation draw your knees closer to your armpits while your hips stay grounded on the floor. This action should come from your hip muscles softening and releasing rather than pulling on your legs with your upper arms and shoulders. Visualize the backs of your hips lengthening from your lower back to your tailbone, and imagine that they are broadening along the floor.

Happy Baby lengthens the sacral joints. It is often a good stretch when pain is present because the hips and lower back are supported by the floor, which allows them to release tension while in a supported and balanced position.

Free-Your-Sacrum Pose

Stretch | Dwi Pada Apanasana Variations

Lie on your back with your legs straight down on the floor. Lift your knees into your chest, holding the backs of your thighs or your shins with both hands. Though I don't often get into the particulars of the poses' Sanskrit names in this book, I want to pause a moment to look at a word that appears in both this pose and the next one: *apanasana*. If the word sounds familiar, it's because I talked about the apana vayu, the downward, grounding energy of the lower abdomen and hips, in chapter 2. Similarly, Apanasana grounds and brings freedom to the whole pelvis. Stay in your base position for three or four breaths. With each exhalation, bring your knees a little closer to your chest while keeping your back hip bones grounded on the floor. Visualize the layers of myofascia around your hips and buttocks broadening and lengthening, then relaxing into the support of the earth.

The following variations are great if your sacral band or lower back feels tight, but they may be contraindicated for strained sacral joints or overly flexible sacral ligaments.

Variation 1: Partner-Assisted Leg Press

Start with both knees bent into your chest with your arms by your sides. Have a partner stand facing you with her knees slightly bent. Ask your partner to place her hands on your shins while you lift your tailbone slightly upward, releasing your sacral joints and lower back into the floor. Press your legs up into your partner's hands while she presses gently down. The push through your legs and your partner's hands should be equal—you are not trying to push your partner away (fig. 3.4). If this feels comfortable,

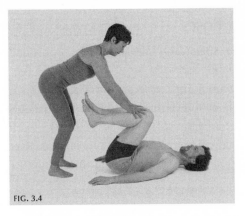

FIG. 3.4

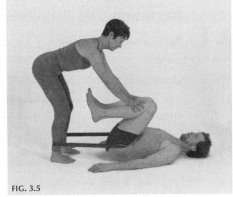

FIG. 3.5

both of you can increase the pressure. Hold this position for fifteen to twenty seconds and release. Rest while you check in with your sacral band to feel how it has opened—it should feel comfortable and soft. Repeat the leg press two more times, and feel how it spreads and broadens the sacral joints.

Variation 2: Partner-Assisted Sacrum Traction

Start in the base pose, then make a large loop in a belt and place it around your front groins, the crease where the very tops of your thighs meet your hips. Have your partner stand facing you with knees slightly bent, and have her step into the belt. The belt should be around the top of your partner's ankles or slightly up along the calves; the belt should be parallel to the floor. If it's possible, position yourself so you can reach your arms all the way over your head and hold onto something heavy, such as a post or a heavy piece of furniture, to create as much traction in your sacral joints as possible.

Now have your partner gently hold your legs in place (no pressing down this time) while she presses her legs backward and walks slowly back, each small step gently increasing the traction along your sacral joints (fig. 3.5). If the belt digs into your front groins, place a folded towel or blanket between the belt and your groins.

Poses that use traction are excellent for freeing compressed sacral joints and lengthening the lower back. Rest with your hands on your lower abdomen when you are done, gently massaging your hips along the floor. Feel energy circulating a little more freely now that your muscular body has released some of its holding, and feel that your hips and sacrum are more spacious.

Reclining Sacral-Balancing Pose

Balance and Strengthen | Eka Pada Apanasana Varaiation 2

Once you've loosened up your sacral joints in Free-Your-Sacrum Pose, you're ready to work on balancing them, one leg at a time. This pose has two steps, each of which helps your sacrum in a different way. Practice both steps two or three times on your right side, resting for a few breaths after each cycle, then repeat on your left side an equal number of times.

Step 1: Bent-Leg Sacral Balancer

Lie on your back with your knees bent and feet flat on the floor, and bring your right thigh to your chest. Lift your tailbone slightly up toward the ceiling while your hips stay grounded on the floor. Stretch your left leg down onto the floor. If you have discomfort in your right sacral joint, try placing a folded blanket under your hips. If you have discomfort in your lower back, place a rolled-up towel underneath it. Hold your right shin or behind your thigh with both hands. Press your right thigh away from your chest until your arms are straight (fig. 3.6), and press your hands equally back into your thigh. Hold your leg in position using the equal pressure of your leg and your arms.[7] Your leg, abdominal core, and back hip muscles should all feel active and engaged as you create traction in your body without the help of a partner.

Move your right outer hip and right sit bone toward your left foot (your right foot can move slightly to the left to help initiate these actions). Hold the position for fifteen to twenty seconds, then release the muscular effort of your leg, arms, abdomen, and hips, and as you exhale, draw your knee toward your chest. This pose, while subtle in its movements, helps to bring your right hip bone and sacral joint into balance and can help your sacral band to feel softer and more spacious. Repeat the pose on your left side. A word of caution, though—if your lower back is tight and this exercise creates compression and pain, release it and move on to step 2.

Step 2: Raised-Leg Sacral Balancer

Bring your right thigh as close as possible to your chest, and hold the back of your thigh with both hands. As in step 1, stretch your left leg straight

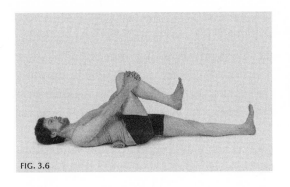

FIG. 3.6

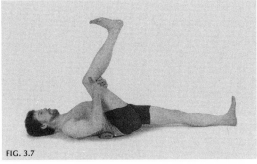

FIG. 3.7

onto the floor. However, this time your arms should stay bent. Hold your thigh close to your chest while you slowly start to stretch your right leg up toward the ceiling (fig. 3.7).[8] You may not be able to completely straighten your leg; that's not as important as holding your thigh in position close to your chest. As you press up into your hands, lengthen your right hip away from your waist. Lift your left leg about three inches from the floor (but keep it active and straight) in order to feel your right hip bone tip back. Maintaining the position of your right hip, slowly place your left leg back down and see if your hips can remain in place. Repeat this step two more times.

This pose helps move a forward-rotated hip bone back into place, and helps to realign your sacral joints as it does so. If your hips are already balanced, practicing this pose on both sides will bring stability into your sacral joints. After you've practiced both steps, repeat the sequence on both sides. As well as balancing your hips and sacral joints, this pose helps relieve pain and release tension in your lower back.[9]

Reclining Hand-to-Foot Pose

Stretch | Supta Padangusthasana I

Now that you've balanced your sacral joints, you're ready to take the next step and stretch each leg straight up toward the sky. This pose lengthens your hamstring and hip muscles. If you have discomfort in your lower back when you bring your knee into your chest, try placing a small rolled towel under your lumbar region.

Bring your right knee into your chest and place a belt around the arch

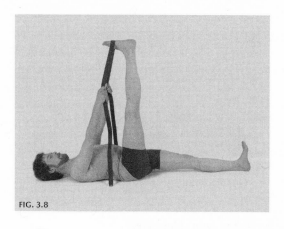

FIG. 3.8

of your foot. Hold the belt with both hands, straighten your arms, and slowly stretch your leg up toward the ceiling (fig. 3.8). Straighten your leg completely by engaging all the muscles of your leg, and imagine hugging your inner knee with your kneecap. Press the center of your arch up into the belt, making your foot parallel with the ceiling. If your hamstrings are tight, lengthen the distance between your foot and your hands along the belt, lowering the angle of your leg relative to the floor. Roll your left leg slightly inward and stretch it away from your torso. Engage your abdominal core by drawing your frontal hip bones up toward your ribs, keeping your hips grounded on the floor.

Right now you may be feeling a huge hamstring stretch and wondering what this pose has to do with your sacrum. Stick with it! Lengthening your hamstrings and deep hip muscles is one of the best things you can do for your sacrum because when your hamstrings are tight, they tug on your hip and lower back muscles and create misalignments and imbalances in your sacral joints. It's always worthwhile to take the time to lengthen your hamstrings. When you do, you will discover a sense of fluid movement and ease all through your hips and spine.

In Reclining Hand-to-Foot Pose, and in the variations described below, remember to move your right outer hip and right sit bone toward your left foot just like you did in Reclining Sacral-Balancing Pose. This action will help bring your hip bones into balance. Be mindful to keep your sacral joints flat and resting on the floor. If you have discomfort in your lower back, place a rolled towel beneath it.

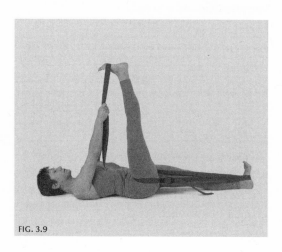

FIG. 3.9

Variations: Supported Sacrum Release

Place a looped belt around the top of your right thigh at your front groin and raise your right leg into the base pose. Ask a partner to stand behind your right leg facing you, and to take

98

the belt around the top of his right ankle or up along his calf, so that the belt is parallel to the floor. Hold your right foot with another belt, or have your partner hold your foot in place, raised toward the ceiling as it was in the original pose. Ask your partner to press his lower leg into the belt and step back, one small step at a time, as you stretch your leg up toward the ceiling and draw your foot toward your head. Feel your hamstring muscles releasing, and feel your sacral joints flat and grounded on the floor.

This partner assist relieves pain due to compressed sacral joints because it creates traction in the sacral joint on the lifted leg side, even more than when you do the pose yourself.

If you don't have a partner handy, you can do this variation on your own by using a long belt looped around your right front groin and your left foot as shown in fig. 3.9.

Hold Reclining Hand-to-Foot Pose and its variation for thirty to forty-five seconds on each side, then rest in Happy Baby Pose (page 93) for a few moments.

Reclining Tree Pose

Balance and Strengthen | Supta Vrkshasana

Reclining Tree Pose helps the sacral joints come into balance. It is most helpful for a sacral joint that is rotated backward, because in the lying-down position, the action in your bent-leg hip will lift the joint upward and help it to come into balance with your other sacral joint. If your sacrum is already in balance, the pose helps brings stability to the joints. I've described it starting on the right side, but you can start on your left if you know that your left sacral joint is rotated backward. Regardless, it's well worth practicing this pose to both sides because of the firmness it brings into the whole sacral band.

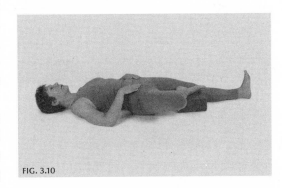

FIG. 3.10

Start by lying on your mat with your legs stretching straight away from your torso. Bend your right knee and bring your right foot to rest along your inner left thigh, supporting your outer right foot on a block so your hips stay even and balanced on the floor (fig. 3.10). Place your hands on your hip bones and balance your hips so they are an even distance from your waistline. Keeping your hips on the floor, lift your tailbone slightly upward and engage your abdominal core muscles. Now engage your right buttock muscles and feel your right hip lifting up toward the ceiling while your buttock stays grounded. This action helps lift the right sacral joint up to the level of your left sacral joint. Hold for ten seconds and relax. Repeat two more times to the right, then practice on the opposite side.

When you are done, rest with your legs down on the floor or with your legs in Reclining Knee Squeeze (page 93) and place your hands on your lower abdomen. Close your eyes and visualize your sacrum as the grand meeting place in your body through which energy now flows easily and with vitality.

Table-Balance Pose

Balance and Strengthen | Vyaghrasana Variation 1

Begin on all fours with your hands under your shoulders and your knees under your hips. Gaze down toward the floor. Keeping your spine in a neutral position, draw your navel toward your spine and draw your frontal hip bones toward your ribs to engage your abdominal core muscles. On an exhalation extend your right leg back and up until it is parallel to the floor. Press your right hand down and stretch up through your right arm, making it stable and strong. With your next exhalation, lift your left arm up and hold it parallel to the floor (fig. 3.11). Firm your deep hip muscles, draw your tailbone slightly down toward the floor, and keep your navel moving toward your spine.

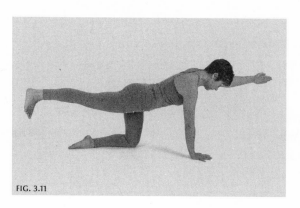

FIG. 3.11

Hold this position using the lift and strength of your abdominal core and your deep hip muscles. Remain for fifteen to twenty seconds, or come down as soon as you feel tired. Rest for a few moments in Child's Pose (page 61), and then repeat with the opposite arm and leg. Table-Balance Pose will help stabilize your sacral joints and strengthen your abdominal core, helping to bring your sacral joints into balance.

Supported Deep Lunge Pose with Variations

Stretch and Strengthen | Virabhadrasana I Variations

Stand two to four inches away from a wall, facing it, and place your hands on the wall, slightly higher than waist height. Cup your hands so just your fingertips touch the wall. Bend your knees and as you exhale, take a big step back—five feet if possible—with your left foot. Keep your left toes pointing straight forward, with your heel up in the air. If you feel unstable or vulnerable, place a folded blanket under your left heel for support.

Now drop your right hip and thigh toward the floor, bending your knee into a deep lunge. As your hip and thigh muscles open and strengthen with time and practice, your right hip will drop so your thigh is parallel to the floor. In every stage of descending your right hip down into a deep lunge, protect your knee joint by making sure your right knee is directly over your right ankle from side to side and front to back. Make sure your left leg stays straight and strong.

Take your left hand onto your sacral bone. Draw both thighs toward your hips—you should feel your sacral joints coming into balance. Just to make sure your hips are even with your sacral joints, draw your left hand around to your outer left hip and encourage it to press forward toward the wall. Support this action by rolling your left thigh inward. Now take your fingertips back to the wall to help support your torso in an upright position, seeing if you can maintain the sacral balance you've achieved.

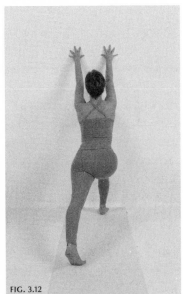

FIG. 3.12

Drop your tailbone down and scoop it toward the wall. Feel how this action creates lift all the way up through your torso and helps keep your lower back elongated. Exhale your navel back toward your spine and feel your abdominal wall supporting your torso. Stay here for a few breaths and see if your lower back is comfortable. If it is compressed or strained, lean your torso forward toward the wall until it releases.

Feel your inner left leg elongating from your sit bone all the way to your inner heel, and lift the back of your left knee up toward the ceiling. Feel the length you are creating along the front of your left thigh as your quadriceps (front thigh muscles) and psoas (the muscle mainly responsible for creating neutral and upright hip position) stretch and elongate. Hold your pose for fifteen to twenty seconds and then come out by straightening your right leg and stepping your left leg forward to meet it. Come back to your starting position at the wall, and repeat the pose with your left leg forward and right leg back.

After you have done Supported Deep Lunge Pose to both sides, you can add two variations to your repertoire. When you have practiced this pose a number of times in complete comfort, you are ready to try Proud Warrior Pose in the "Grow and Progress" section of this chapter , page 119.

Variation 1: Sacral Broadener

Come into Supported Deep Lunge Pose with your right leg forward and your left leg back. Turn your left toes inward so they are facing slightly to the right, turning your left heel slightly out to the left. Reach through your left leg strongly from your sit bone to your heel, as if you were trying to ground your heel (your heel should not touch the floor, though). This foot position creates more internal rotation in the left hip joint, which in turn creates more stretch in your piriformis muscle and more broadness across your sacral band. Be sure not to drop your left hip down; hold your hips in as much balance as possible. Reach your arms as high up on the wall as possible (fig. 3.12). Hold this position for ten to twenty seconds. Then stand tall in Mountain Pose for a few moments, close your eyes, and experience the sensations in your left thigh and hip before repeating the pose to your opposite side.

Variation 2: Grounding Lunge

Starting in Supported Deep Lunge Pose with your right leg forward and left leg back, turn your left toes slightly outward this time, so your left heel descends to the floor.

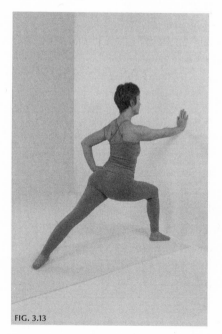

FIG. 3.13

YOGA FOR A HEALTHY LOWER BACK

Notice whether your left hip rotates backward when you place your heel down. If it does, mindfully reposition your left hip so it faces forward (fig. 3.13). Remember to drop your tailbone toward the floor to elongate your sacral joints and lumbar spine.

Keeping your spine as upright as possible and your head level, place your hands on the wall. Feel your body moving in two different directions at once—the base of your hips descends down toward the ground while the rest of your body lifts from your hip bones up through the crown of your head, creating an uplifting movement in your spine. Come out of the pose as before, and repeat with your left leg forward and your right leg back.

Protect Your Sacrum: Tips for Healthy Backbends

The next three poses are backbends that will strengthen your lower back and lengthen your psoas muscles. Earlier in this chapter, I described why backbends are good movements in a healthy sacrum, and now I want to teach you some specific actions that will help your body feel comfortable while you practice them.

If you have sacral issues, you may have been told backbends can help. Prone backbends including Cobra and Locust Poses are often the first yoga poses suggested by physical therapists for lower back pain. The theory behind the practice is clear and logical—those poses strengthen the buttock, hip, and lower back muscles, and elongate the psoas and front thigh muscles. All these actions contribute to your body's ability to carry its weight through your lower back and sacral joints. But if not practiced with care and support, back-bending movements can exacerbate back pain. You can experience the benefits of prone backbends *and* avoid discomfort by following a few "rules" for how to move your body in these poses. Keep the following in mind for the next three poses, and whenever you practice a backbend lying on your front body:

- Ground your front body firmly from your feet up to your abdomen whenever your legs are positioned on the floor.
- Stretch your legs and torso away from your waist to create length for your back.
- Bring your hips to neutral position, and draw your tailbone down toward the floor while you engage your buttock muscles. Your buttock muscles should be firm (but not tightly gripped) so your sacral joints feel stable.

- Lengthen your frontal hip bones toward your waist. You will feel this action as you draw your tailbone down, but if you are unsure, place your fingers on your frontal hip bones, and draw them up your body. You will feel length in your front groins and thighs.
- Remember what we learned earlier, that your sacral bone nutates—it naturally moves forward toward your front body as your spine comes into a backbend. You can help create room for your lower back to move into a backbend comfortably by consciously elongating your lower back and waist forward before lifting them up into a back-bending position.
- If the floor creates discomfort in your frontal hips, lie on a folded blanket.

Supported Cobra Pose

Strengthen | Salamba Bhujangasana

Lie on your front body and place a bolster or two stacked, folded blankets crosswise in front of you. Place your forearms on the bolster and draw your torso right up to the bolster. As you move, engage your buttock muscles while you draw your tailbone toward the floor; engage your leg muscles and abdominal core. Press your forearms down and lift your torso up so your breastbone is high and your collarbones are wide (fig. 3.14). Imagine you

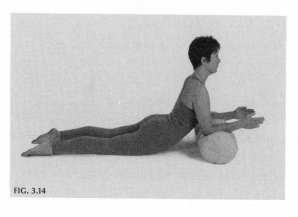

FIG. 3.14

are able to lift your heart higher than your breastbone. Draw your shoulder blades away from your ears and press them forward to help support your chest. Pressing your forearms on the bolster helps elongate and lift your spine, especially at the meeting place of your sacral and lumbar spines, where it tends to overarch and compress in traditional Cobra Pose. If your sacral band feels achy, practice the pose without the bolster, placing your forearms and hands on the floor and lifting your torso up only as much as is comfortable in your lower back.

Supported Cobra Pose is very therapeutic for weak or imbalanced sacral joints. The support that the actions of your buttock muscles and abdominal core provide helps to draw your sacral joints toward your front body and "reset" them into a balanced position. It feels particularly soothing if you have sprained your sacral band. If your body likes Supported Cobra, hold it for a few minutes.

Your body will tell you when it is time to come out of Supported Cobra Pose. If your back starts to ache or feel compressed, it is time to release the pose. Move the bolster away from your body and rest with your head on your hands for a few breaths. Bend your legs, point your toes up to the ceiling, and sway your shins from side to side, feeling gentle movement come into your hips and sacral band. Press your hands into the floor and lift your shoulders and hips up, coming onto your hands and knees. Then move into Child's Pose (page 61) for a few breaths.

Alternate Arm/Leg Prone Backbend

Strengthen | Shalabhasana Variation

Lie on your front body with your legs and arms stretched away from your torso. Place your feet about hips' distance apart and place your hands shoulders' width apart. Rest the center of your forehead or your chin on the floor, whichever is more comfortable for your neck. Place a pillow under your abdomen if your lower back is uncomfortable.

Press your tailbone down toward the floor and firm your buttock muscles. Feel your hips balanced and equally grounded. As you inhale, lift your right leg up while keeping your hips even. Press your right hand down into the floor and lift your left arm and shoulder up (fig. 3.15). Stretch your right leg and left arm away from

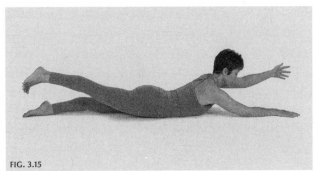

FIG. 3.15

each other, creating as much length along the diagonal of your body as you can. Keep your hips grounded on the floor—no tipping to one side or the other. Hold for about fifteen seconds and release your leg and arm down. Repeat three or four times on the same side, rest for a few breaths, and repeat the pose an equal number of times on your opposite side. When you are done, fold your forearms and rest your forehead on your hands.

The muscular work of lifting your right leg and left arm goes directly through your right sacral joint, stimulating and strengthening the myofascia around the buttocks while your hips are in a supported, stable position. Energetically speaking, this work goes directly through the Svadhisthana (sacral) chakra, stimulating and strengthening the first meeting place of the Ida, Pingala, and Sushumna energy channels through which Kundalini flows. Be mindful not to turn your lifted toes and foot in or out; reach your big toe and little toe equally away from your hips.

Supported Locust Pose

Strengthen | Salamba Shalabhasana

Lie on your front body with your arms stretched out in front of you and a chair or stack of blocks within reach. Press your hips and legs down and lift up your arms, one at a time, placing your hands on the lower support rung of the chair or blocks. Press your hands down on the prop while you lift your shoulders, trunk, and head upward. Draw your torso forward any amount possible so you feel your lower back lengthening as it moves into a backbend (fig. 3.16). Your whole back body should feel engaged in this pose; be sure your tailbone keeps pressing down

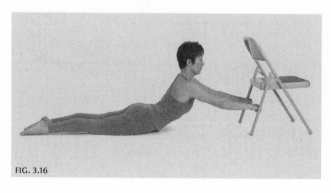

FIG. 3.16

so you are elongating your lower back. If it's completely comfortable, increase the stretch to your spine by placing your hands onto the seat of the chair, or you can add more blocks to your pile, but be sure your lower back does not feel compressed. Hold the pose for fifteen to twenty seconds and slowly release, bringing one hand at a time back down to the floor.

YOGA FOR A HEALTHY LOWER BACK

When prone backbends such as Supported Locust Pose are practiced with mindfulness and attention, they are excellent for toning the musculature throughout your lower back. This pose can be soothing for imbalanced sacral joints, and it can give them stability to move through day-to-day activities and carry the weight of the middle and upper back.

Forward-Bending Hero's Pose

Stretch | Adho Mukha Virasana

Although Forward-Bending Hero's Pose appears similar to Child's Pose, it is quite different because it is an active, if neutral, stretch for your spine, while Child's Pose is a passive resting position. After practicing backbends, it's good to rest in a forward bend—and we will—but it's even better to stretch out your spine in a neutral position first. Remember that the sacral bone naturally goes into the movement called nutation when you do a backbend; following that motion with the counternutation of a forward bend is an important balancing action. Before you start, review the notes about sacral counternutation on page 79, and refer to page 88 to review how forward bends release your sacrum.

Variation 1: Active Pose

Kneel on a mat (or a blanket if your knees hurt) with your knees about hips' distance apart, and bring your toes together. Sit down on your heels. If you can't sit on your heels, place a folded blanket or bolster between your calves and thighs. Place your hands on the mat in front of you, and walk your hands away from your trunk, keeping your arms active, elbows lifted off the ground, and the front of your trunk elongating (fig. 3.17). Reach your breastbone as far away from your hips as you can so the front and back of your trunk are both long. Be mindful not to overarch your lower back upward or round it downward. You can grip the floor with your fingertips and crawl your arms farther forward, giving yourself a nice stretch in your shoulders as well as along your back. When you can't reach your trunk any farther forward, stay for a few breaths, giving your spine time to release.

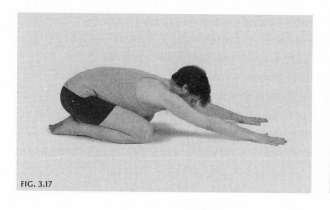

FIG. 3.17

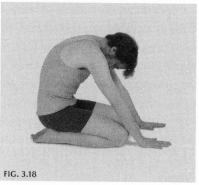

FIG. 3.18

Variation 2: Resting Pose

Now you can give your back a soothing forward bend release. Starting in Forward-Bending Hero's Pose, lift your trunk and shoulders and walk your hands closer to your hips. Be sure to keep your hips grounded on your heels or on a folded blanket. Place your hands flat on the floor and actively push the floor away from you while you drop your tailbone down toward the floor. Your navel will move back toward your spine (fig. 3.18). You should feel a gentle stretch in your lower back, and your sacrum should feel relaxed. Now take your arms by your sides and turn your palms upward. Rest your arms, shoulders, and head on the floor for fifteen to twenty seconds. Support your head on a block if it doesn't reach the floor. Relax completely.

Half Forward Bend Pose

Stretch | Ardha Uttanasana

If your sacral band felt comfortable in Forward-Bending Hero's Pose, you're ready to try a standing forward bend, which can be more challenging because your sacral band won't be supported on your thighs. We'll start with Half Forward Bend Pose to make sure forward bending works for your sacrum.

Stand tall facing a wall with your feet about hips' distance apart. Place your hands on the wall at hips' height. Bend your knees and mindfully walk your feet away from the wall until they are directly under your hips. Keep

YOGA FOR A HEALTHY LOWER BACK

your knees bent while you lift your sit bones up toward the ceiling, and elongate the front of your trunk forward toward the wall. Roll your upper thighs inward to deepen your groins as you feel your hips folding over your thighs. As much as possible, your back hips should be parallel to the floor so your sacral joints are even with your hip bones. Draw your shoulder blades away from your neck and look forward, lengthening your breastbone and collarbones toward the wall (fig. 3.19). Stay in this modified forward bend for a few breaths, feeling the fold at your hip joints,

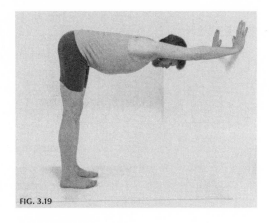

FIG. 3.19

the length of your torso, and a sense of comfort and stretch in your sacrum.

Slowly stretch your legs straight one at a time, as you did in the forward bend experiment we practiced earlier in this chapter on page 88. Keep your sit bones lifting, and be sensitive to any shifts in your hips and lower back. If your sacrum is comfortable, stretch your legs completely straight, otherwise keep a slight bend in your knees so you don't overround and strain your sacral joints or your lumbar spine. Try turning your toes inward to feel even more broadening of your sacral band.

Come out of Half Forward Bend Pose by bending your knees and walking toward the wall. Keep your hands at the wall until you are once again standing upright.

If Half Forward Bend Pose at a wall is comfortable for your sacral band, try a slightly deeper version by placing your hands on the seat of a chair and walking back into the pose until your hips are right over your feet and your trunk is long. You'll enjoy more stretch all along your back body and a deeper bend at your hips.

Standing Forward Bend Pose

Stretch | Uttanasana

When Half Forward Bend Pose is comfortable for your sacrum, you can practice full Standing Forward Bend Pose.

Stand with your feet hips' distance apart with your legs, trunk, and

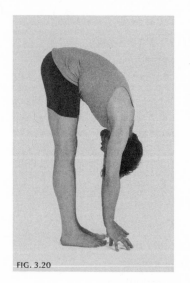

FIG. 3.20

spine elongating upward in Mountain Pose. Place your hands on your hips and fold from your hips, drawing your trunk first forward and then toward the floor. While moving into the pose, place your hands on your thighs for extra support and bend your knees slightly to make folding at your hips easier. Place your hands on the floor (fig. 3.20), or on blocks or a chair if they don't reach the floor. Take your trunk down only as far as your sacrum very comfortably allows. Slowly straighten your legs. Remember to turn your upper thighs inward, and your toes too, if that was a good feeling in Half Forward Bend Pose, to help spread your sacral joints.

Standing Forward Bend elongates all the muscles of the back body, and it's especially helpful for releasing a tight sacral band. If your sacral joints are weak or imbalanced, proceed with caution. You'll want to keep the back of your hips in alignment as much as possible, bend your knees, and pay special attention to lifting your sit bones upward as you fold forward. This will help your sacral joints follow the forward movement of your hips so your lower back holds its integrity as you bend.

Stay in Standing Forward Bend Pose for a few breaths. Let your hamstrings release any amount possible, and enjoy the feeling of your back body stretching from your heels, over your bent hips, and all the way through the crown of your head. Softly inhale, and come out of the pose with your hands on your hips or thighs, whichever is more comfortable for you. Stand with your eyes closed for a few moments and visualize the energy at your Svadhisthana and Manipura chakras stimulated and alive through the massage they just received. Visualize the webs of your sacral ligaments and the musculature of your back hips opening and "breathing," drinking in fresh energy from your rejuvenated chakras and a wash of fresh blood to help them become healthy.

Variation: Decompressing Forward Bend

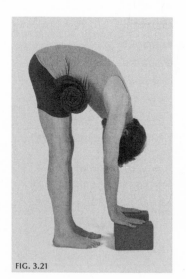

FIG. 3.21

Hold a rolled blanket or a bolster along the top of your thighs. Folding your trunk at your hips, come into Standing Forward Bend. Release your arms toward the floor, placing your hands on blocks, or hold your elbows and let your arms descend.

YOGA FOR A HEALTHY LOWER BACK

Your front ribs should rest on the roll (fig. 3.21). If they don't, or if the roll slips toward the floor, bend your knees until you can hold the roll between your thighs and trunk. This is soothing and relaxing for sacral compression because it gently elongates the musculature of the back of the hips and the lower back.

Restorative Twist Pose

Rest | Parshva Balasana

Sit on the floor with your legs straight forward. Lean to your right, bend your knees, and shift your shins and feet to your outer left hip. Rest your hips evenly on the floor. If you have a knee or hip issue that stops you from resting both hips on the floor, sit on a folded blanket. Separate your knees and let your legs relax.

Place a bolster at a ninety-degree angle to your right hip. Place your hands on either side of the bolster and gently turn your torso to the right so it is centered on the bolster. Now lay your torso down onto the bolster. Turn your head to the right, to give your neck a gentle stretch, and relax. Let your arms rest along the floor.[10]

Ahh . . . that should feel good! This is a restorative pose, which means that your body is receiving a gentle, opening stretch in a completely supported position. In other words, right now you have no work to do; just let your body completely let go and relax (fig. 3.22).

Breathe into your sacrum and feel it broaden. Breathe into your spinal muscles and feel them gently elongate along the bolster, bringing your spine into a soft twist from your lower back all the way up to your neck. You can turn your head to the left if that makes your neck more comfortable. Stay in Restorative Twist Pose for as long as you are comfortable, then come out by pressing your hands into the floor to lift your spine up. Swing your shins over to the right side of your body, move the bolster to your left side, and repeat the twist to your left.

Restorative Twist Pose gently stimulates your whole lower back. The myofascia

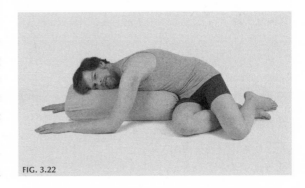

FIG. 3.22

releases along diagonal lines, lengthening the deep hip musculature and the webs of ligaments that cover your sacrum—imagine being able to hold a spider's web and gently elongate it diagonally. The Ida, Pingala, and Sushumna, the energy pathways we've discussed throughout this chapter, are opened and stimulated in this pose, resulting in an easy, unrestricted flow of energy from the Muladhara chakra at the base of your hips all the way up your spine to the Sahasrara chakra at the crown of your head. No wonder this pose feels so nourishing and enlivening!

Deep Relaxation: Rest into the Earth

Rest | Shavasana Variation 2

Now it's time to completely let go and rest your sacrum into the support of the earth. You'll need a bolster, one or two folded blankets, and a rolled towel. Have your eye pillow handy if you like to rest your eyes.

Place your bolster across your mat and sit behind it. Drape your legs over your bolster so it is directly under your knees. Lie back onto your elbows and press your forearms down into the floor to elongate your trunk. Slowly, vertebra by vertebra, rest your upper body onto your mat (or a blanket for an even softer experience). Slide your hands under your upper thighs and buttocks and draw them out to the sides to create the feeling that your sit bones and sacral joints are spreading apart from each other. Let your feet rest with your toes pointing slightly outward (fig. 3.23). Be sure your heels are resting on the floor; place a folded blanket underneath them if they are not.

If your lower back is uncomfortable when you lie down in this position, try one of these variations and see if you can find the support it needs to relax:

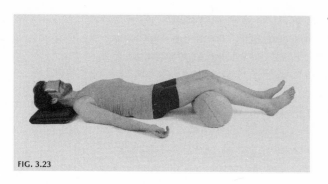

FIG. 3.23

- If your sacral joints feel loose or weak and your sacrum feels too "flat" against the floor, place a rolled towel under the top of your sacral band, adjusting the height of the roll for comfort. This gives direct support to your lower back, helping the muscles and myofascia to relax and restoring your lower back's natural, gentle curve.

YOGA FOR A HEALTHY LOWER BACK

- If your lower back feels tight or compressed, place a folded blanket under your hips. This elongates your lower back.

After you've gotten into a position of absolute comfort in your sacrum, rest your head on a folded or rolled blanket. Place your eye pillow gently across your eyes, feeling your eyes calming down and softening inward. Finally, rest your arms on the floor, angled slightly away from your body so your shoulders roll gently down into the support of the earth. Rest your palms facing up or down, whichever is more comfortable for you.

Relax your throat and neck, and feel the center of your skull resting into your mat or blanket. Let go in your jaw, feeling it slightly open, and release your facial muscles out to the sides of your face and down toward the floor. Take time here and use a few breaths to move your attention from the body's outermost layer, your skin, to the deep layers of your facial muscles; you will feel your face losing its everyday expressions and becoming neutral and passive. Creating a feeling of neutrality in your body will help your mind come away from its attachment to thoughts so it is neither pulled toward positive thoughts nor pushed away from negative ones. Feel your mind becoming balanced and centered, a witness to thoughts without judging or being affected by them. Feel your mind becoming impartial to what it finds as it observes your body, and ready yourself to go even farther inward in meditation.

In the Yoga Sutras of Patanjali, sutra 1.33 states, "The mind becomes clear and serene when the qualities of the heart are cultivated: Friendliness toward the joyful, compassion toward the suffering, happiness toward the pure, and impartiality toward the impure."[11]

Take a few minutes to meditate on these qualities and how they live in your heart. When your mind moves into a neutral state, you can look within and see what exists there without making a judgment about yourself. Can you find friendliness, compassion, happiness, and impartiality toward yourself? Now, can you direct these qualities toward your tight, overstretched, weak, or achy sacrum? Cultivating these qualities can help you deal more easily with discomfort and pain—in your sacrum and beyond. That's one big benefit. Another is that once you treat yourself with friendliness, compassion, happiness, and impartiality, you can engage with the world surrounded by those same qualities. Yoga practice helps you live comfortably in your own body and engage with others with a benevolent, serene countenance.

Visualize friendliness, compassion, happiness, and equanimity growing in your heart. Rest with your attention in your heart for a few moments, until your mind and heart become united in these qualities. With your next exhalation, visualize serenity flowing from your heart deep down into your sacrum. Hold your awareness in your sacrum now, and feel that with each breath peacefulness moves throughout your sacrum, cleansing and rinsing away tightness, holding, darkness, and dullness—all the toxic things that can settle into the sacrum and cover its light.

Now visualize that sacral light, the subtle, coiled Kundalini energy, awakening and flowing through your sacrum and through the energy channels of your spine, bringing life and energy into every part of your being.

Grow and Progress

Once you are comfortable with all the poses in the practice section, you are ready to move on to practice poses that require more stability and strength in your sacrum. I've included a few poses that ask for more stretch across the sacral band and a few that build strength in your lower back—excellent next steps for moving forward in your sacral healing journey. I've also included seated twists, which some students with sacral issues love and which completely vex others. The twists are sequenced starting with less stretch and moving into deeper stretch. Start to practice them slowly and explore how they feel in your body. In particular, proceed into Proud Warrior Pose and Wide-Legged Standing Forward Bend only when you feel confident that your sacral joints are ready to do so. You'll know when you're ready because you'll be able to describe your sacrum with the quote from the Yoga Sutras of Patanjali that I mentioned in chapter 2: *sthira-sukham asanam*, which means that a posture should be "steady and comfortable."[12]

Chair-Seated Twist

Stretch | Bharadvajasana Variation

For this pose, you'll need a folding chair, or any chair in which you can sit with your knees level with your thighs and your feet flat on the floor. Sit with the right side of your body parallel to the back of the chair. Place your feet directly below your knees, and place a block between your knees. Your feet should be even with each other and so should your knees. Place your hands on your hips and feel that they are balanced over your legs. Squeeze your knees into the block to hold it in place; this stabilizes your hips and sacral joints.

With an inhalation, lift your arms straight up. As you exhale, turn your torso to your right and place your hands on the back of the chair. Press down on the chair with your hands to help lift your torso upward as you inhale, and gently push your left hand into the chair to turn more deeply to the right as you exhale. Be mindful that you are rotating your torso and not your hips. Keep your torso as upright as possible, and keep the centerline of your head aligned with the center of your sternum. Once you've moved into a comfortable twist, with your lower back in a sustainable stretch, turn your head to the right and glance over your shoulder to give your neck a gentle stretch (fig. 3.24). Caution, however, is advised for those with neck issues.

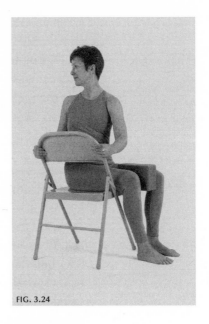

FIG. 3.24

I've started this section with Chair-Seated Twist because it is an excellent way to rotate your spine and elongate your lower back while keeping your sacral joints and hips aligned and stabilized, which makes it safer for imbalanced sacral joints than poses in which your hips are freer to move around. Twists can feel particularly soothing for a sacral sprain or if your lower back feels compressed. If your sacral joints feel overstretched, experiment with placing a belt around the widest part of your hips to create stability in the joints.

Seated Crossed-Legged Pose Flow

Stretch | Gomukasana Variations

You practiced Reclining Crossed-Legs Pose in chapter 2, giving the piriformis and gluteus maximus muscles a good stretch while your sacral joints and lower back were supported on the floor. Now that you are ready to go a little deeper into your hips and sacrum, you'll practice a seated version of this pose with a twist, side bend, and forward bend added in. Seated Crossed-Legs Pose may feel like a strong stretch in your hips and across your sacral band. I have two suggestions that might help you do it safely and fully—the first is to sit up on as much height as you need so you feel a comfortable, sustainable stretch, and the second is to take a break between each of the four steps listed below. Come out of the pose, stretch your legs, even walk around the room once or twice, then come back into the sequence until you have finished all four steps.

Step 1: Cross Your Legs

Sit with your legs extended straight forward. Bend your knees and fold your left shin under your right leg. Then cross your right leg over your left leg. Bring your knees as close to one another as you can. Be sure your hips are in an upright, neutral position. Sit on a bolster or a folded blanket if this is difficult or if there is discomfort in your hips or your knees (fig. 3.25). Stay here for a few breaths and let your hips release. Visualize your hip bones spreading and wrapping around your outer hips, and visualize your sacral joints broadening and expanding. As the backs of your hips spread, visualize your frontal hip bones moving gently toward each other, creating a feeling of softness in your lower abdomen.

Step 2: Twist Your Spine

Like Chair-Seated Twist, this is a good twist for those who are dealing with sacral issues, because your hips and sacral joints are firmly stabilized by the position of your crossed legs.

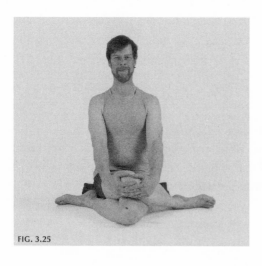

FIG. 3.25

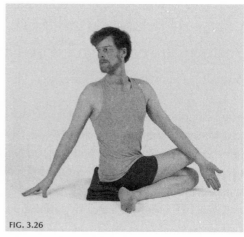

FIG. 3.26

YOGA FOR A HEALTHY LOWER BACK

Starting in the position described in step 1, lift your arms up with an inhalation and elongate your entire spine upward. As you exhale, turn to your right. Place your right hand on the floor (or on a block if you are sitting on a prop) behind your hips and place your left hand on the outside of your right thigh with your arm straight. With each inhalation lift your spine upward and, if your sacrum is comfortable, deepen the twist each time you exhale.

The key to happiness in any twist is to move mindfully—and if you have a sacral issue, be sure your sacrum is stable and your spine is twisting gently from the bottom up. Slowly twist your lower back and waist first, then your ribs, then your upper chest and your shoulders. Let your head just follow along with the turning of your spine so you move from your core rather than your neck or head. When you've reached your final twist position, turn your head to look over your right shoulder and toward the floor, completing the twist through your entire spine (fig. 3.26). If you have a neck injury, though, keep your nose and chin in line with your breastbone.

Slowly unwind your spine and release the twist. You'll twist to your left when you change the cross of your legs. Right now, move on to the side-bending step described below.

Step 3: Bend to Your Side

In Seated Crossed-Legged Pose (step 1), place your left hand on the floor about a foot away from your left hip. Lift your right arm up and over your ear, leaning to the left as long as the right side of your trunk feels a comfortable stretch (fig. 3.27). For more stretch, you can place your left forearm on the floor. Breathe into the musculature along your right hip, waist, and ribs and let your side body release as you exhale. Hold the stretch for fifteen to twenty seconds, then press your left hand into the floor to help lift your torso back up to sitting position.

Side bending stretches the outer hip, the sacral band, and the lower back. After you come out of the pose, sit upright for a breath or two and bring your awareness into your right hip. Feel length and space along the sides and back of your hips and across your sacral band.

Step 4: Bend Forward

Start again in Seated Crossed-Legged Pose. Lift your arms up over your head with an inhalation, and as you exhale, bend forward from your hips,

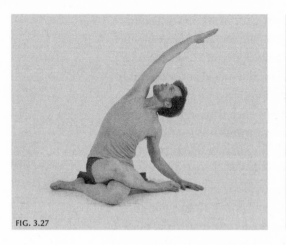

FIG. 3.27

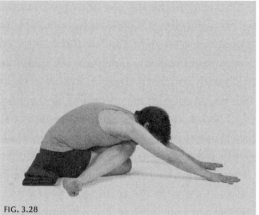

FIG. 3.28

placing your hands on the floor in front of you. If you can't reach the floor, place your hands on a block. As you inhale, elongate the front of your trunk upward, and with your exhale start to move into a forward bend (fig. 3.28).

It's important to feel that your spine is moving forward as you come into a forward-bending position, even though your sacral joints will naturally move slightly backward in counternutation. You can tell if you're on the right track by placing your hands on your back hip bones. As you bend forward, can you feel your back hip bones also moving forward? If so, you're bending correctly, from your hips rather than from your back or chest. From your initial bend, let your lower and middle back follow your hips and sacral bone into a gentle, even curve along your whole spine. If your hip bones and lower back collapse backward, though, place your hips on more height until you feel the difference.

Hold the pose for fifteen to twenty seconds. Bring lots of breath into your hips! Feel the back of your hips and your sacral band broadening and expanding, remembering what you've learned about the sacral bone's healthy counternutation movement. Slowly come up from the forward bend with an inhalation, and return to Seated Crossed-Legged Pose.

After completing all four steps, change the cross of your legs and repeat the sequence. You should experience spreading across your whole sacral band, because this pose is particularly helpful for relieving tightness and tension in your sacrum.

Proud Warrior Pose

Stretch and Strengthen | Virabhadrasana I

Before you attempt to practice Proud Warrior, a strong standing pose that builds stamina while it expands stability and power in your hips and spine, be sure your body feels very comfortable in the Supported Deep Lunge Pose with Variations on page 101.

Stand in the center of your mat and step your feet about five feet apart. Turn your left toes slightly inward, and turn your right foot and leg ninety degrees to the right. Place your hands on your hips and turn your hips and torso to face your right leg. Balance your waist, chest, and shoulders from left to right. Place one hand on your lower abdomen and the other on the back of your hips. Drop your tailbone toward the floor and lift your hip bones up toward your chest, bringing your pelvis into the upright and neutral position that I described in the Low Lunge Pose (page 51).

Draw your shoulder blades down and away from your ears and press them forward, transforming them into hands that support and open your front chest (we'll talk more about this in chapter 6). On an inhalation, lift your arms up over your head, keeping your front chest broad. With your next exhalation, bend your right knee and drop your right hip toward the floor (fig. 3.29). Hold your left leg with strength so you have power in both legs to support your body. Look forward, or if you feel very stable, look up, letting your head dip behind your arms. Stay in the pose for fifteen to twenty seconds, and come out by reaching your arms even more strongly upward and straightening your right leg. Turn your feet in the opposite directions, and repeat Proud Warrior Pose on your left side.

To alleviate any feelings of compression in your lower back, make sure your arms, ribs, and waist are all lifting upward; if you still have discomfort, lean your torso forward to make length in your lower

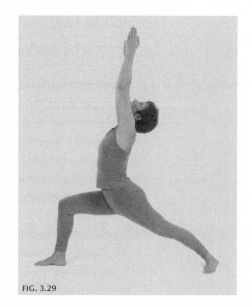

FIG. 3.29

back. But perhaps the best way to create comfort in your sacrum, hips, and lower back in Proud Warrior Pose is by maintaining neutral hip position throughout the pose. Be sure your tailbone is consistently dropping down toward the floor and scooping slightly forward, your hip bones are lifting upward toward your chest, and your navel is moving back toward your spine. Be sure to draw both your thighs toward your hips, as you did in Supported Deep Lunge Pose with Variations, so that your sacral joints come into balance.

In this challenging but empowering pose, breathe deeply down into your torso and visualize your Svadhisthana (sacral) chakra. Imagine this vital energy as your center of gravity and stability, expanding and supporting your sacrum through its strength. Breathe up into your chest and feel your heart becoming expansive and open. As your breath moves between your lower and upper torso, visualize the energies of prana vayu and apana vayu joining and uniting, creating an energetic oneness in your body. Feel a self-supportive sense of personal power and a sense of oneness as your parts unite.

Allow yourself to feel proud of your body for gaining the strength and flexibility to move comfortably through this pose.

Wide-Legged Standing Forward Bend

Stretch | Prasarita Padottanasana

After a strong pose like Proud Warrior, it's good to let your body rest for a few moments, but in a position where you can enjoy the feelings of strength and tone you've created in your legs, hips, sacrum, and spine. Wide-Legged Standing Forward Bend is just such a pose. In steps 1 and 2 you'll feel your spine lengthen and let go of tension and tightness, and as you move into the final step, your mind will have a chance to quiet down and experience the flow of energy in your spine.

Stand on your mat with your feet four to five feet apart, with a pair of blocks at the midpoint between your feet, slightly forward of your body. Feel your feet evenly grounded into the floor, and be careful not to collapse your ankles inward or overstretch them outward. Lift up through your legs, as if you were drawing the supportive energy of the earth all the way up your legs into your lower back. Bend forward from your hips and place your hands on the blocks, making sure your hips stay aligned with your ankles so you don't tip forward.

Step 1: Half Wide-Legged Forward Bend

Lift your torso halfway up, elongating your waist, the sides of your trunk, and your lower back. Your torso should almost be parallel to the floor (fig. 3.30). If your spine is unable to lengthen in this manner, place your hands on the seat of a chair instead of blocks. Stay here for a few breaths and observe how lifting energy up through your legs stabilizes your body and helps you lengthen your trunk away from your hips, releasing tightness and tension in your lower back. Gaze forward if your neck is comfortable. You can increase neck comfort by drawing your shoulder blades away from your neck. If your neck is in discomfort, look down at the floor.

Step 2: Half Wide-Legged Spine Lengthener

With the next few exhalations, move your blocks or chair away from your body, reaching with your arms and elongating your torso and your spine. Keep your hips directly over your ankles so your lower back gets the benefit of gentle spinal traction. Your trunk will be at an angle to the ground now—the farther you reach your arms and trunk forward, the closer your shoulders will come toward the floor (fig. 3.31). Hold this stretch for a few breaths while your spine reconfigures to a new length.

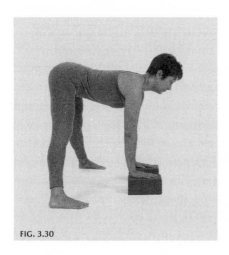

FIG. 3.30

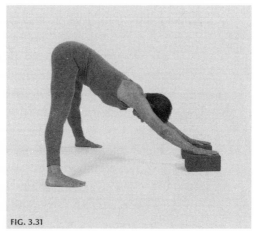

FIG. 3.31

Step 3: Full Forward Bend

Release your props and walk your hands along the floor back toward your body, until they are in line with your feet. Release your trunk, shoulders, and head straight down toward the floor. Rest the crown of your head on the floor, on a block, or even on a pile of blocks, however you can allow your head to connect to the earth. Visualize the supporting energy of the earth flowing up through your legs and hips, into your trunk and spine, with each inhalation. Feel your lower back relaxing and releasing, energy pouring freely along your spinal muscles from your sacral joints to the nape of your neck (fig. 3.32). Visualize the central channel of your spine, the Sushumna, as a luminescent core of energy around which Ida and Pingala dance, and where they come together at each chakra, visualize points of light that illuminate your path to wellness.

Although Wide-Legged Standing Forward Bend isn't an inversion (in an inversion, your legs are higher than your heart), it gives you some of the restful benefits that inversions offer: The easy flow of blood from the torso to the heart, because it is aided by gravity in this pose, signals the heart to beat slower and reduce the strength of its contractions.[13] Further, the stimulation of the vagus nerve (we'll talk about this more in chapter 5) in a head-down position elicits the relaxation response of the parasympathetic nervous system.[14]

To come out of the pose, come back into step 1 by walking your hands under your shoulders and lifting your trunk halfway up. As you start to come up, be sure to listen to your sacrum, which has been given an awakening, enlivening yogic experience. If it is happy, come up with your hands on your hips, your legs strong, and your spine lifting straight up. But if you sense any discomfort across your sacral band, place your hands on your hips, bend your knees slightly, and slowly roll your spine up to a vertical position. Walk your feet together and stand tall in Mountain Pose for a moment. Feel your whole back body filled with freely flowing energy that travels from your feet up along your back all the way to the crown of your head before sinking back down into your feet, grounding you to the earth.

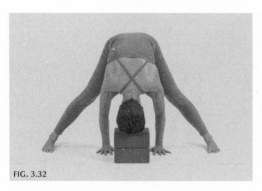

FIG. 3.32

YOGA FOR A HEALTHY LOWER BACK

Child's Pose and Deep Relaxation

Rest | Balasana and Shavasana Variation 2

It's important to completely rest your body after every practice, and that's especially true when you are exploring more rigorous poses such as those in this section. Rest in Child's Pose (page 61) for one to two minutes and then in Deep Relaxation, as described on page 112, for as long as ten minutes if you have the time. Support your sacral band for absolute comfort and let your body completely relax into the support of the earth.

4

Your Lumbar Spine

If the sacrum is the "heart" of your spine, then the five vertebrae that make up your lumbar spine form a major "artery" carrying nourishment, energy, and support up from your core, through your trunk, and toward your upper body.

Like the sacrum, the lumbar spine is a chronically neglected region of the modern human body. The word itself sounds tight, stiff, and clumsy. (Confession time—did you ever think it was spelled "lumber"?) You've no doubt noticed—and possibly invested in—the industry offering "lumbar support" pillows for planes, trains, and automobiles, your desk chair at work, or a night at the movies. If you're among the millions of Americans who has visited a doctor complaining of "back pain," chances are your lumbar spine has been part of the problem.[1]

The reason for this is that the lumbar region has a lot of work to do. Most of your body weight is borne by its musculature, and most of the movement your back is capable of comes from this area of your spine. All this responsibility can leave your lumbar spine vulnerable to injury and strain.

Unless, of course, you know how to take care of it, which is where the yoga practice in this chapter comes in. When it comes to the lumbar spine, the physical work in yoga is to create as much balance as possible while respecting and honoring structural conditions and limitations. In this chapter you will explore your own lumbar spine, and with yoga, you will create your body's natural tone and balance.

THROUGH WESTERN EYES: THE PHYSICAL VIEW

Close your eyes and visualize your pristine lumbar region, the area of your back between your hips and the bottom of your back ribs. The muscles on either side of your spine are long, smooth, and gently curved inward toward the front body. They are evenly developed; the right and left sides are balanced. There is a slight indentation between the spinal muscles that forms a "valley" where the spinous processes—the knobby, bony protuberances that extend backward from each vertebra—are just visible. Imagine touching your lumbar muscles and feeling how pliable they are, how they yield to your touch, and how they return to their original shape when you take your fingers away.

Wait . . . is this not your experience with your lumbar?

In reality, the lumbar muscles can be visibly—and painfully—imbalanced, with one side thicker and wider than the other, or, in the case of a hip imbalance or variations in leg length, one side longer or shorter than the other. The muscles can be curved and wavy, as in the case with a scoliosis. Sometimes there's no "valley" between the muscles at all, and the spinous processes press too far outward, forming a line of foothills climbing uncomfortably up the back. In other bodies, the valley is so deep, the lumbar muscles so overly thick and stiff, that one can barely see the skin, much less a hint of a spinous process. Some lumbar spines have a reverse, convex curvature. If your back is strongly imbalanced and you come into a standing forward bend, your lower back can look like a buckled and collapsed road after an earthquake, not a smooth, rolling highway on a clear day. I have seen all these conditions in my students' lumbar areas.

Looking through the lens of Western medicine, let's start with bones, muscles, and ligaments. Your lumbar spine (illustration 13) is composed of five bones, the L1-to-L5 vertebrae, which sit between your middle and upper back—called the thoracic spine—and your sacral spine. The lowest lumbar vertebra, L5, sits in between your back hip bones, where it connects with S1, the top sacral vertebra.

The joint between L5 and S1 allows for the rotation of your hips when you walk and run. This joint, along with the one above it, between lumbar vertebrae L4 and L5, are the most weight-bearing joints of the lower back. Consequently, they are the most prone to stresses that cause injury. More on the challenges associated with L5/S1 in a moment.

Unlike its neighbors, the sacral spine and the thoracic spine, your lumbar spine is a flexible stack of bones. Remember that your sacral bone is grounded into your back hip bones, so its range of motion is limited. Your thoracic spine is connected, by your ribs, to your breastbone, so it too is relatively limited in its options for movement. By contrast, there are no bony structures in your lumbar region to limit its movement in healthy, supporting ways, except at the very bottom, where L5 resides between your back hip bones.

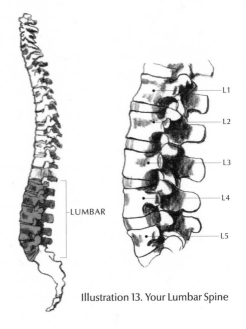

Illustration 13. Your Lumbar Spine

Sit in a chair for a moment and see if you can feel what I mean. Move your shoulders and upper chest around, feeling movement throughout your shoulder girdle and chest. Feel how your whole upper chest, back, and shoulders are connected and moving together, unified by the musculature and bones that surround the area.

Now move your hips around on the seat of the chair, feeling how your sacral bone and hip bones are connected to one another and move as a unit, again stabilized by the musculature and ligaments around them.

Moving both your hips and your upper chest, now feel your lower back and visualize your lumbar spine. Feel how much movement there is in your lumbar region and around your waistline. Unless your back is extremely tight, you are probably feeling a lot of movement!

When I experience the movement of my lower back this way, I visualize that I'm holding a pearl necklace vertically with one hand holding each end. The pearls dangle and move as I move my hands, staying connected by the strong but supple threads that link them. Like this imaginary pearl necklace, the lumbar vertebrae are connected to each other by ligaments, the spongy intervertebral disks (commonly simply called "disks"), and the spinal muscles, which give it tremendous strength and allow for increased mobility, but there's not a lot else there to restrict its movement. It's as if your lumbar spine could do a dance all its own—swaying, bending, and twisting, unfettered and fluid. To offer a second image, you can note that the spinal nerve roots that travel through the lumbar and sacral spine, branching out into the lower body, have the Latin name *cauda equina*, because of their resemblance to a horse's flowing tail.

The chain of pearls and the horse's tail are beautiful, graceful images for unencumbered, fluid movement and spaciousness in your lower back and abdomen, but you'll only experience them if your lumbar and abdominal core muscles are strong and the myofascia is flexible, working together to support your lumbar spine while it moves around. It's the job of the musculature to help the bony structures of your entire body move in a coordinated and healthy way, and that may be even more important in your lumbar region because of its independent nature. If the lumbar muscles are imbalanced, if your hip bones are tilted, if you have different leg lengths, or if some muscles are strong and others are weak, the vertebrae of your lumbar spine can get pushed and pulled around until injury happens to the lumbar ligaments, muscles, or the spinal disks themselves. The vertebrae can shift out of alignment with one another, putting pressure on the disks and the nerves that run through the spinal column to the abdominal organs, hips, and lower legs.

The fact is, lower back injuries and conditions are almost as common in our culture as the common cold. According to the National Institutes of Health, they are second only to the cold as a reason for a visit to the doctor.[2]

But I would argue that "lower back pain" is too general a term. The types and intensity of lower back injuries and conditions are numerous and include arthritis, ligament and muscular strain and tears, a narrowing of the spinal canal (spinal stenosis), degenerative disk disease, spinal curvature (scoliosis), nerve root compression, slippage of one vertebra forward of the one beneath it (spondylolisthesis), herniation and rupture of the spongy disks between vertebrae, and an inflammatory arthritic condition that mainly affects the joints between spinal vertebrae (ankylosing spondylitis).

The therapeutic use of yoga for these conditions varies greatly from condition to condition. I do want to mention again that if you have had persistent pain for over two weeks and/or numbness, tingling, or weakness in your hips or legs, a diagnosis by a medical professional is of the utmost importance prior to beginning a yoga practice.

The Lower Lumbar Challenge: L4, L5, and S1

As we explore the lower back, it's important to understand that the most vulnerable part of the area, and the most common place of injury, is where your lumbar spine meets your sacral spine.

There are two main reasons why. First, as I mentioned earlier, the joint between the top of your sacral spine at S1 and the base of your lumbar spine at L5 is extremely important—and equally vulnerable. For one thing, it is the lowest joint in the spine that includes a spinal disk, since the sacral vertebrae below it are fused together. When the lumbar spine bends forward, backward, or to the side, or when it rotates in a twist, the sacral spine stays in position with minimal movement. You can imagine the stress this can place on the disk between S1 and L5.

Second, you'll remember that lumbar vertebra L5 sits nestled below the top of your back hip bones in your sacrum, while L4 sits just above those bones. L5 doesn't move that much, because it is connected to the back hip bones by the iliolumbar ligament, which stabilizes the pelvis when you bend to the side. Sometimes this ligament extends up to lumbar vertebra L4, but in most bodies it does not. You're probably already imagining why the joint between L5 and L4 is so prone to injury: L5, wedged snugly inside the pelvic girdle, doesn't have as much movement as L4. So if you overwork your back in a side-bending, lifting, or twisting action, L4 moves and L5 doesn't necessarily move along with it. This creates stress and strain in the ligaments around those vertebrae, leaving the disk between them particularly vulnerable to injury. Snow shoveling, anyone? Gardening? Your lower back might be aching just thinking about it.

For these two reasons and others, injuries to the disks in the lower back are quite common. A disk becomes "herniated" when all or part of the spongy cushion inside it is forced through a part of the disk that is weak, either due to repetitive or sudden, jolting movements that cause stress and strain.[3] A herniated disk can eventually rupture, releasing spinal fluid and causing severe pain.

I talked a little about sciatic nerve pain and piriformis syndrome in chapter 2. Thinking about how common the diagnosis of "sciatica" is, it's probably not a big surprise to learn that the nerve fibers that bundle together to form your sciatic nerve come out of the area of your spine between lumbar vertebra L4 and sacral vertebra S3, right at the intersection

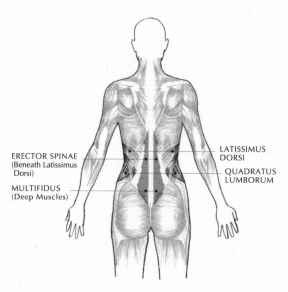

ERECTOR SPINAE
(Beneath Latissimus
 Dorsi)

LATISSIMUS
DORSI

QUADRATUS
LUMBORUM

MULTIFIDUS
(Deep Muscles)

Illustration 14. The Muscles of the Lower Back

of your lumbar and sacral spines, where the lumbar spine is most vulnerable to injury.[4]

A diagnosis of sciatica or "radiculopathy" may also be given in the case of pain that radiates from the lumbar region through the hip and down the leg along the path of a spinal nerve root. These conditions can be caused by compression, inflammation, or injury to a spinal nerve root arising from a number of conditions, including a herniated disk, spinal stenosis, degenerative disk disease, and spondylolisthesis.[5]

In case you haven't had enough anatomy yet, here's a quick sketch of the major lower back muscles (illustration 14), all of which will figure into the yoga practice in this chapter:

- The latissimus dorsi muscles, the big, broad outermost muscles that wrap around from the thoracic and lumbar spines to the side chest and the upper arm. Although this muscle group's main role is to move the shoulder joint, it also participates in the extension and lateral flexion of the lumbar spine.
- The erector spinae group, which bends your spine backward (extension), contributes to side bending (lateral flexion), and supports your spine in the upright position.
- The transversospinalis group, especially the multifidus muscles. These short, often overlooked major postural muscles help your lumbar spine extend and twist. They are what connect vertebra to vertebra all the way up your spine, and they remain in contraction for long periods of time while the spine is moving, standing, and sitting. Weakness in the multifidus muscles is common to many types of lower back pain.
- The quadratus lumborum muscles, which connect the lumbar spine from L1 through L4 to the back hip bones on either side of the spine and allow the lumbar spine to bend sideways and backward. Spasms of the quadratus lumborum muscles are a common source of lower back pain.

The tone of your hamstring muscles, which you felt when you experimented with a simple forward-bending exercise (page 88), also has a major effect on the health of your lumbar region; if your hamstrings are tight, they can tug on the hip bones, which in turn pull on the muscles of your lower back, potentially flattening the natural inward (lordotic) curve of your lumbar spine and creating stress and misalignments in your lower back.

Your psoas muscles are also important players in the game of lower back health because those muscles are involved in both forward bending (flexion) and the rotation of your trunk. If one or both of your psoas muscles are tight, they can pull your lumbar spine forward and down toward your lower abdomen. The lower back muscles then become contracted; the result is an uncomfortable exaggeration of the natural curve of the lumbar spine called *lordosis*. In this extreme position, the lower back can take on a form diagnosed as "swayback posture."[6]

Lordosis might not sound so bad in and of itself, but it has a ripple effect up through your spine that can open up a world of tension and imbalance. Your body is always working toward balance, and if your lower back is out of whack, everything else adjusts to "balance" around it. The middle and upper back does this over a lordosis by overrounding backward into a position called *kyphosis*, which is an exaggeration of its natural outward (kyphotic) curve.[7] Then your neck gets in on the act, overarching forward and bringing your head with it. Once your head is forward of your shoulders, all manner of tightness erupts in your neck, upper back, and shoulders, contributing to chronic upper back pain, as well as headaches and migraines. This is one of the best examples I can think of to illustrate the interconnectedness of all the parts of your spine—an action deep in your back (tight psoas muscles) has an effect all the way up into your head.

Before we move on to the Eastern view of the lower back, a brief note about the abdominal core is in order. Although I will spend much more time in chapter 5 on the abdominal core muscles, it is helpful here to know that the muscles of the anterior abdominal wall (what you typically refer to with the general term "abs") support your lumbar spine by maintaining pressure on its concave curve. They help the entire spine to bend forward, and when they are toned, they can actually help resist the tendency of the lower back muscles to form an exaggerated lordosis. So when you create support for your lumbar spine with your abdominal core muscles, you counteract not only excessive lordosis but—because everything in the spine is interconnected—excessive thoracic kyphosis and neck contractions as well.

Because of its remarkable interconnectedness, the lower back responds to what's happening below it in the legs, hips, and sacral spine, what's happening in front of it in the abdomen, and what's coming down into it from the head, neck, and middle and upper back. In fact, the lower back and the neck have a very deep connection with each other, because they share the same concave curvature. An injury to the neck, such as a whiplash or a head injury, can have a direct effect on the health of the lower back as well.

In this chapter you will practice yoga poses to strengthen and tone the musculature around your lumbar spine. When you start to practice, decide if a pose feels good, both while you are in it and when you come out of it. If it feels good, it's a keeper! But if you start to feel pain in a pose, do not move more deeply into it; listen to your body's feedback and practice only what helps you to feel better. As your lower back becomes more toned and strengthened, you will be able to expand your repertoire to include a broader range of poses.

THROUGH EASTERN EYES: THE ENERGETIC VIEW

I often receive e-mails from students after yoga classes. One student wrote that her lower back had never felt better than it did the morning after our class. Another student wrote that he gained new insight about how to take care of his lower back and, with his pain lifting, he had more positive energy to use in various aspects of his life. When I looked back at the practice sequences for the particular classes the students were referencing, I realized that the sequences had just what a hurting lower back needs. In them, we practiced a good balance of spinal elongations, backbends, twists, forward bends, and deep relaxation. In doing so, we not only physically massaged and toned the lumbar area, we massaged the energy of the third (Manipura) chakra and activated points along the nadis called *marma* points, which distribute prana to specific parts of the body—in this case, the lumbar.

Chakras: The Fiery Power of Your Lumbar Spine

Your lower back and abdominal area is the home of the Manipura chakra, the energetic center of vitality and personal power that includes the area around the navel and the solar plexus. In chapter 3, I noted that the activation place for the Manipura chakra is right behind your navel, which is aligned with the top of your sacral spine (illustration 15). You've now learned that the top of your sacral spine is the meeting place of the sacral and lumbar spines. So as we look through Eastern eyes at the lumbar spine, we've come right back to the L5/S1 area that I called "the lower lumbar challenge"—the most vulnerable part of the lower back.

The flip side of this vulnerability, though, is the potential for great power and strength. When balanced and strong, this area is an active, powerful location in the body, full of creative possibilities, self-activation, inner power, heat, and fire—both energetically and physically.

The Manipura chakra encompasses the area between your navel and your diaphragm; it is the home of the "fire in the belly" of Western psychology, the passionate readiness to fight with energy and determination for what you believe is ethical and right. In yogic terms, it is the home of *agni*, the fire of transformation that fuels the digestive system and burns up energetic impurities, cleansing the subtle layers of your body and releasing residue with each exhalation. It is often depicted with red and yellow hues, true to its fiery nature.

Manipura is a magnificent source of energy and personal power—the good kind of power that helps you to forge good relationships with others and helps you direct your creative energies into positive actions.

An image traditionally associated with the Manipura chakra can help you understand the immensity of its power—the image of the sun. The power of the Manipura comes from the presence of solar energy residing there, just as the term *solar plexus* in Western anatomy implies.

Even though the chakras don't have direct physical locations in the body, we are always encountering the interconnected overlay of the physical and energetic bodies. In a holistic view, the energy of the chakras makes impressions on their corresponding physical areas, and the energy of your physical body in turn imprints on the energetic areas. If either the physical or the energetic body isn't functioning smoothly, the other may be affected.

Marma Points: Vital Centers of Energy

In the system of traditional medicine native to India called Ayurveda, there are points

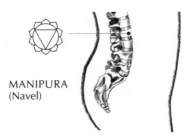

MANIPURA
(Navel)

Illustration 15. The Manipura Chakra

associated with the nadis, the energetic channels we discussed in chapter 3 (page 83). These are called *marmani,* or marma points. These points are connected with specific anatomical areas of the body, but they are much more than that. In their book *Marma Points of Ayurveda,* Vasant L. Lad and Anisha Durve define marma points as "vital energy points infused with prana, where consciousness is most expressive."[8] Marma points are a bridge that spans the body, mind, and soul. They are similar to the acupuncture points that Traditional Chinese Medicine teaches run along the energetic meridians of the body. The difference between the two is that marma points are located on the surface of the body rather than deeper within, where acupuncture points reside. And many marma points are located directly on their associated anatomical areas, which makes them highly accessible and easy to use for therapeutic purposes. Similar to Western massage techniques, marma point therapy loosens knots in the physical body, and similar to acupuncture treatments, it releases blockages and brings balance to the energetic body.

Ayurveda hypothesizes that activating marma points with massage and pressure facilitates cellular communication, cleanses and rejuvenates the physical body, and calms the mind and emotions. Marma point treatments support the body's balance and healing ability by increasing the flow of prana through the nadis, bringing balancing and healing energy into the targeted area. Marma point therapy is used in Ayurvedic medicine to treat everything from elbow pain to neurological conditions, as well as for a full range of internal-organ disorders. Due to the lack of research on Ayurveda in the West, this system has not been integrated into conventional medical treatment plans. However, as knowledge about Ayurveda increases, it is finding a place in Western health care and contributing to better health and well-being.

How do marma points relate to your lumbar spine? Very much so, especially three "sets" of points:

- *Kukundara* points (Sanskrit for "that which supports the spine") are located right where your lumbar and sacral spines meet, on each side of lumbar vertebra L5.[9]
- *Kati* points, meaning "hip or waist," are located just below the lumbar spine, at the openings in sacral vertebra S1, one of the locations from which the sacral nerves emerge.[10]

- *Vrukka* points, meaning "organ of water filtration," refer to your kidneys. These points are located between lumbar vertebra L1 and the thoracic vertebra T12 on each side of the spine.[11]

UNITING EAST AND WEST: THE HOLISTIC VIEW

The Kidneys and Your Lumbar Spine

Looking through a holistic lens, an interesting connection between your physical and energetic bodies is how your lower back interacts with your kidneys and adrenal glands, and how these glands affect your energetic well-being. Your kidneys sit squarely inside your lower back, between thoracic vertebra T12 and lumbar vertebra L3, and they play a critical and unique role in the body's overall health. From a Western viewpoint, they are essential in the urinary system, they help regulate blood pressure, and they filter and remove waste from the bloodstream, among other things. The adrenal glands sit on top of the kidneys and regulate the production of the hormones adrenaline and cortisol, both of which are released by stress and participate in the fight-or-flight response of the sympathetic nervous system. Of course, we need the fight-or-flight response in critical situations, but it's an intention of yoga practice and Eastern medicine to bring the fight-or-flight response into balance with the relaxation response of the parasympathetic nervous system so the energetic body comes into a state of equilibrium and health.

In Chinese medicine, a concept that is analogous to prana is chi or qi (pronounced "chee"). The kidneys are considered by the Chinese to be the regulators of life force, balancing yin and yang, rest and activity. Kidney chi regulates the overall state of energy in the body. And here we encounter another correlation between East and West: in Chinese medicine the emotion of fear is associated with the kidneys and adrenals; in Western medicine, fear signals the adrenal glands to release adrenaline and cortisol.

From a holistic perspective, when the lower back musculature is tight or injured, the kidneys and adrenals may become compressed and stagnant, which in turn can affect your vitality, overall sense of well-being, and ability to relax.

Students have told me that they feel afraid to move when they have lower back pain, thinking they will worsen the injury. Did you catch the word *afraid* in this common response to lower back pain? Understanding and calming fear is unquestionably part of the process of healing your lower back, as Dr. John E. Sarno's 1991 bestseller *Healing Back Pain*, among other books, argues.[12] I encourage these students to practice gentle twists, backbends, and forward bends, all of which tone the lumbar musculature and massage the kidney area. I also suggest breathing techniques that elicit the relaxation response of the parasympathetic nervous system though elongated breaths and deep exhalations. Ocean Breath, which you learned in chapter 1 (page 12), is an excellent example of this, especially when you practice it using extended exhalations.

I also encourage them get an Ayurvedic treatment that includes activation of the marma points in the sacral and lower back areas, to help stimulate the functions of the kidneys and adrenals. Soon, students' backs start to feel better and their fear goes away. Their bodies are more comfortable, and their minds are calmer.

As we begin this chapter's exercises, create a supportive intention for your practice. Practice for the health and happiness of your lower back. Meet your lower back where it is with mindful, curious, nonjudgmental attention. Accept that your lower back may not be able to do all the exercises now, but that the poses might be possible for you to practice in the future. Listen to your body's feedback about which poses feel good to your lower back, and practice them whenever you can. Over time, your lower back will surely become a place of tone and vitality.

Yoga Poses for a Healthy Lumbar Spine

Ask and Listen: Preparation for Practice

Almost all back-injury therapies rely on stretching and strengthening movements to help heal lower back pain, but passive rest is also an essential, therapeutic part of healing. It helps release tightness in the superficial back muscles, brings circulation and prana into an area of restriction or injury, and creates a dialogue between you and your back so you can start to understand it. We will end our practice as always with deep relaxation, but let's also begin it with a calming, meditative check-in with your lumbar spine.

Reclining Lower Back Meditation with Ocean Breath

Fold one blanket lengthwise and lay it down on your mat. Sit in front of the short end of the blanket with a few inches between the blanket and your hips. Bend your knees and place your feet flat on the floor. Place your hands on the floor behind your hips and slowly lie down, elongating your entire spine as you do so. Support your head on a second folded blanket. Take time to scan your body, especially your lower back, and make sure it's completely comfortable. If it is, straighten your legs along the floor and relax (fig. 4.1).

If your lower back isn't comfortable, however, lie down as you did in Deep Hip Meditation (page 42) with your back flat on the floor, your knees bent and your feet flat on floor. Support your neck and head for extra comfort.

Direct the flow of your breath down through your chest into your lumbar spine and all the way into your hips as you inhale, and let it softly flow up from your hips to your chest as you exhale. Let it energetically caress and massage your lower back. Visualize your psoas and lower back muscles releasing tension and relaxing with each breath. Simply rest here for a few moments with mindful focus on the flow of your breath.

Visualize the flow of prana into your lower back, helping it come into its natural alignment—a long, gentle, natural upward curve free of clenching or muscular gripping.

Deepen the flow of your breath into your lower back by bringing Ocean Breath, which you practiced in chapter 1 (page 12) into your practice on both your inhalation and exhalation. Ocean Breath, you may remember, is a soft, resonant, vibrational breath that comes from gently constricting the back of your throat.

When you practice it in this pose, remember the rule of thumb I use for breathing in my classes: "soft breath for a soft pose, strong breath for a strong pose." Since this is a soft pose, create a subtle, soft vibration in your breath. Feel your deep inhalations lengthening and

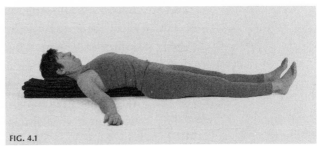

FIG. 4.1

expanding your lower back, elongating the muscles, increasing the mobility in your joints, and gently stretching the myofascia. Visualize the soft, resonant vibration of your exhalation moving deeply into the muscle fibers, untying the physical knots in your muscles and allowing them to absorb fresh, new energy.

As long as your body is comfortable, stay in Reclining Lower Back Meditation for five to ten minutes so you experience some therapeutic rest. Maintain Ocean Breath for as long as your breath's rhythm is smooth and soft. If your breath hardens or if you feel tension anywhere in your body, release Ocean Breath and rest in the pose with normal breathing.

Reclining Crescent Moon Pose

Lie on your back with your arms reaching over your head; take your hands all the way to the floor if you can. Engage the muscles of your legs and reach them away from your trunk. Your knees should face the ceiling and your feet and toes should point toward the ceiling. This is Reclining Upward Hand Pose.

Keeping your legs active and long, draw them to your left. Hold your right wrist with your left hand, and with an exhalation, draw your arms over to your left. Your shoulders, upper back, head, and hips should all remain on the floor. Reach your arms and legs as far to the left as both sides of your torso comfortably allow (fig. 4.2). Breathe into the right side of your waist and explore how this gentle stretch feels in your lower back. You will feel length in the muscles on the right side of your back and a gentle contraction on the left side. Use your breath to help open the right side of your trunk and lower back any amount, gently expanding it as you inhale and allowing muscles to release and relax as you exhale. Hold the pose for a few breaths and gently release your right arm. Bring your arms and legs back into Reclining Upward Hand Pose and repeat to your left.

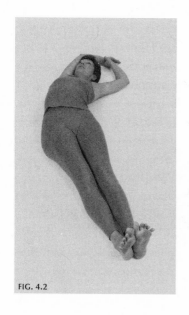

FIG. 4.2

Practice the pose to each side again, this time exploring the similarities and differences on the two sides. Is the stretch even on both sides? Is there more tightness on one side of the lower back than the other? Can you bend equally to the right and to the left, or is one side stiffer? Practicing this pose will give you information about the symmetry (and asymmetry) of your lower back.

If you have scoliosis, you will feel the obvious difference in the two sides due to the rotation of your spine. If you have a disk injury, you may feel that one side of the musculature is much tighter than the other. Even if you simply tend to hold stress and tension on one side of your body, the imbalance in your lower back muscles may be pronounced. Besides being an excellent tool for mindfully understanding your lower back, this is a helpful pose for releasing knots and scar tissue in the myofascia on the elongated side of your body.

Cow-and-Child's-Pose Flow

You practiced Cat/Cow Cycle in chapter 2 as a preparation for Big Hip Circles. In this sequence, Child's Pose takes the place of Cat Pose, because it brings your spine into a similar gentle upward arch in a more restful position. The movement from Cow to Child's Pose also gently massages your hip myofascia and abdominal organs, elongates the spinal muscles, and provides a moment of therapeutic rest before you move back into Cow Pose.

Step 1: Cow Pose

Start in Cow Pose; I'll review it here as a refresher. Kneel on all fours with your hands under your shoulders and your knees under your hips. Support your knees on a folded blanket and/or place a rolled towel under your ankles for comfort. Inhaling, lift your sit bones, collarbones, and the crown of your head upward while you draw your lower back down toward the floor. In this pose, you are bringing your lower back into extension, creating a concave (downward) arch in your lower back that elongates the front of your lumbar spine and its myofascia and increases the space between each vertebra. This allows the intervertebral disks to expand and open at the front of the spine. Move your middle and upper back in toward your front body also, so your whole back moves into *extension*. If your lower back is tight and overarched, take care to move slowly and gently into Cow Pose so you don't overdo the movement. Visualize each disk breathing and becoming a resilient and spongy cushion between the vertebrae.

Step 2: Child's Pose

Exhaling, gently draw your tailbone toward the floor and move your hips down onto your heels. While you move your hips down, draw your navel in and up toward your spine so your lower and middle back come into a gentle convex (upward) curve. Keep your hands in the same place you had them in Cow Pose so your arms and shoulders remain open. Now move into Child's Pose. If you can't place your hips on your heels, or if you have knee discomfort, place a blanket between your calves and thighs.

Now your lower back is in *flexion,* which elongates the back of your lumbar spine and increases the disk space between the back of each vertebra. Inhale into your lower back, visualizing length coming into all the muscles that tend to tighten up and contract. Feel the relief in your lower back as you exhale, your muscles give way, and your spinal muscles release.

See if you can fold forward enough to rest your chest on your thighs—this helps bring space, and holistically speaking, energy into the area around your kidneys and adrenal glands. The flow of fresh blood and prana helps bring the organs into balance, and in turn they help to balance your blood pressure and nervous system.

Step 3: Cow-and-Child's-Pose Flow

Using mindful, deep breathing or Ocean Breath as your guide, slowly move back and forth between Cow Pose and Child's Pose six to eight times. Inhale as you come into Cow Pose and exhale as you move into Child's Pose. This gentle, flowing movement from spinal extension to flexion softens and loosens the lower back muscles. Visualize length and spaciousness coming into that liminal space between sacral vertebra S1 and lumbar vertebra L5 during both movements—along the front of the joint while you come into Cow Pose and along the back of the joint while you move into Child's Pose.

In each movement, let your inner eye travel up your lower back, visualizing each disk, until you reach the top of your lumbar spine at L1. As you mindfully move up through your lower back, notice where it feels comfortable or distressed. Is there one area that feels more compressed? Can you feel where the muscles are tired or weak? Are both movements comfortable, or does one or the other irritate your lower back? If that is the case, lessen the intensity of the movement until your lower back feels comfortable. You will be able to move your spine fully in both extension and flexion as your back becomes more toned and flexible.

Practice for a Healthy Lumbar Spine

Reclining Spinal Twist

Stretch | *Supta Padangusthasana III*

Spinal twists activate the deep back muscles and stretch the connective tissues that help realign and maintain a healthy spine. Begin this twist by coming into Reclining Hand-to-Foot Pose (page 97) lying on your back, lifting your right leg, and holding your right foot with a belt. Now change the hold of the belt so you're holding it with your left hand. Take your right arm straight out to the right, laying it in line with your shoulder. Keep your right leg straight and walk your left hand up the belt until your left arm is straight. As you exhale, draw your right leg over to your left, lifting your right hip up off the floor as your leg twists to the left (fig. 4.3). Go slowly at first and observe your sacrum. If it grumbles or crackles with discomfort, untwist until you are comfortable.

If you can bring your right foot all the way across your body but not to the floor, use a chair or stacked blocks as supports. If your sacrum gives you a "thumbs up" for a full twist, take your right leg all the way over to the left, placing your foot on the floor or on a single block. For a full spinal twist, turn your head to the right, gazing at your right hand.

Enhance your practice by trying the following:

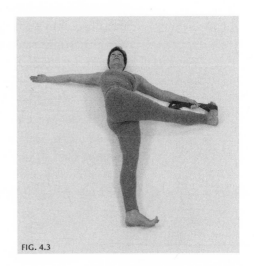

- Place your right hand on your outer right hip, press your hip up into your hand, then draw your hip away from your waist—this lengthens the musculature on the right side of your lower back, and you may feel more stretch along your outer right leg. Breathe deeply into the stretch in your outer right hip and along your outer leg.

FIG. 4.3

- For an even deeper twist—if it's comfortable in your body—press your right hip farther to the left with your right hand.
- Spread your collarbones apart so your right shoulder and upper back remain on the floor and feel relaxed in the twist. If there is tension in either, support your right foot on a higher support.
- Draw the tops of your shoulders down to the floor and draw your shoulder blades away from your neck. Then find the bottom tips of your shoulder blades and gently lift them up toward your front chest to help open and broaden your chest.

Visualize the action of the pose twisting and rinsing your spinal muscles (and your kidneys as well) and as you release the pose, visualize fresh blood and energy flowing into your lower back.

Seated Lower-Back Side Stretch

Stretch | Parshva Sukhasana

Sit on the floor in a cross-legged position. If your knees are higher than your hips, sit on a folded blanket. Take your hands behind your hips onto your sacral joints and be sure they are lifting upright. Elongate your torso, and be sure that your heart area is open and broad.

Place your left hand on the floor about two feet away from your left hip. Exhaling, lean your torso to the left until you feel a comfortable stretch along the right side of your trunk. For less stretch, place your hand on a

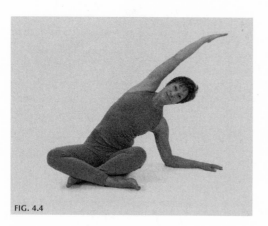

FIG. 4.4

block. For more stretch, place your forearm on the floor, being sure your right hip remains grounded on the floor. Stretch your right arm to the right and turn your palm upward, then reach it up and over your left ear (fig. 4.4). Keep your right arm straight so you actively stretch through your entire right side, from your waist all the way to your fingers.

If you can't sit on the floor comfortably, even on a folded blanket, sit in a chair with your feet about two feet apart. Be sure your feet are flat on the floor. Hold the front edge of the seat with your left hand, lean to your left and stretch your right arm overhead and to the left.

This stretch targets the myofascia and ligaments on the side of your trunk and lower back, especially the quadratus lumborum muscle and the iliolumbar ligament, which are often indicated in lower back pain. Stretching away from the "sore" side, if you have one, often provides immediate relief.

Hold the pose for fifteen to twenty seconds, breathing through the right side of your lower back and feeling it elongating and the tight areas opening and releasing, as if the flood gates of a dam have opened and the right side of your back is once again a flowing river of energy from your sacral joint to the crown of your head.

Extended Puppy Pose and Side Puppy Pose

Stretch | *Adho Mukha Svanasana Variations*

Extended Puppy Pose

This sequence is a prequel to the famous (or infamous, depending on your experience of it) Downward-Facing Dog Pose, known as the "all-in-one" pose because it stretches and tones so many parts of your body at once, including your entire spine. You'll get ready for Down Dog by practicing its younger sibling, Extended Puppy Pose, so you can warm up and stretch your hips, lower back, and shoulders without undue pressure in your wrists and shoulders.

Start on all fours on your mat. Bring your hands to the very front of your mat (yes, that means *all* the way up there!) and walk your feet back to the very back of your mat; curl your toes under. Pad your knees for comfort if needed. Stretch your arms actively, and, keeping your elbows lifted off the floor, stretch your hips backward, away from your shoulders. Lift your sit bones up (fig. 4.5). Your hips should be high in the air rather than descending down toward your feet. Remember,

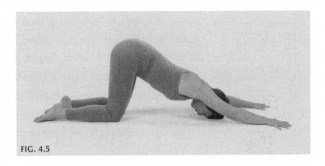

FIG. 4.5

this is not Child's Pose—your pose should feel active in the arms, lower back, shoulders, and sit bones.

Looking forward, move your chest down toward the floor. Now let your forehead rest onto your mat; if it doesn't reach, place it on a block or folded blanket. Breathe through your entire spine and feel a stretch all the way from your lower back up to your shoulders. Visualize your spine lengthening. You can practice Ocean Breath to help deepen the stretch as you inhale and calm your mind as you exhale. Hold Extended Puppy Pose for fifteen to twenty seconds, enjoying the length that comes into your lower back, and the quiet that comes into your mind.

Side Puppy Pose

Start in Extended Puppy Pose. On an inhalation lift your head and shoulders about one foot from the floor and walk your arms over to your right, bringing both arms past your right leg. On an exhalation descend your chest and head down, and also draw your tailbone toward the floor so your hips descend toward your heels. This should feel different from the hip position in Extended Puppy Pose; now you should feel a gentle convex curve in the left side of your back. Keep your arms straight as you reach your arms as far away from your trunk as is comfortable to your left side.

Breathe into your entire left side, starting at your sacral joint, up into your lower back, and through your middle and upper back. Hold the pose for fifteen to twenty seconds, feeling space and length all along left side. On an inhalation, come back into Extended Puppy Pose, then repeat Side Puppy Pose to the opposite side.

A Note About Downward-Facing Dog Pose

Now that you've warmed up your hips and trunk in Extended Puppy Pose, you are ready to explore Downward-Facing Dog. I mentioned before that it's called the "all-in-one" pose. That's because Down Dog, as it is often affectionately called, stretches the entire back side of your body: it brings flexibility into your hips, it tones your legs, and it stretches and opens your entire spine and shoulder girdle. At the same time, it actually rests your heart because when your hips are higher than your heart, the flow of blood from hips to heart moves more easily with the help of gravity. It's one of the best poses you can practice for the health of your whole body, and it's especially good for your lower back.

Yet what I love just as much as the physical stretch in Down Dog is the quiet feeling it brings into students' minds. I can see it on their faces afterward; it's as if a switch to the chatter in their brains has been turned off, and they can draw their awareness deeply inside, letting go of thoughts and distractions for a few quiet moments. This change may be caused by the head's downward position, which stimulates the vagus nerve, eliciting the relaxation response of the parasympathetic nervous system.[13] (See page 175 for more on the vagus nerve and the parasympathetic nervous system.)

Your hips and sacrum are the fulcrum point where all the energy of your body converges in Down Dog. Physically speaking, everything lifts up to this point. You stretch up from your wrists, arms, and shoulders, all the way through your spinal muscles into your sacrum. At the same time, you ground your feet and lift strongly through your legs up into your hips. Energetically speaking, the energy that converges in your hips and sacrum flows back down through your upper and lower bodies, nourishing your musculoskeletal system and internal organs. When I visualize a body in Downward-Facing Dog, I visualize the hips and sacrum as a radiant sphere of energy from which rays of light cascade all through the body to the hands and feet.

First you'll try Down Dog as it is classically practiced. Just in case you don't feel some of the benefits of the pose or if there is too much pressure in your wrists or shoulders, I'll also offer some modifications. Somewhere in this mix, perhaps your mind can find a few moments of peace and quiet.

Downward-Facing Dog Pose

Stretch | Adho Mukha Svanasana

Come onto all fours on your mat. Place your hands slightly forward of your shoulders and place your knees slightly back from your hips. Spread your hands open and feel all your fingers and both palms grounded into the earth. Take a deep inhalation, visualizing your body fill with prana, and with an exhalation, lift your knees off the floor and take your hips up as high as you possibly can. Stretch up from your wrists into your shoulders,

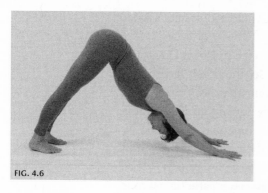

FIG. 4.6

through your trunk, and into your hips. Stretch your legs completely, pressing your thighs away from your trunk and reaching your heels toward the floor (fig. 4.6). Take deep breaths and use the power of your inhalations to lift up through your body. I often tell students, "You can't lift your hips too high in Down Dog!" But in this chapter on the lumbar spine, I want to add a caution: don't raise your hips by overarching your lower back. Your lower back should elongate as much as possible, flowing evenly and smoothly up from your middle back into your hips.

You can play with your legs in Down Dog to create more length in your spine. This is especially helpful if your heels don't reach all the way to the floor in the pose. Try bending one knee and pressing the opposite hip back, elongating that side of your trunk as much as you can. Then change sides, bending the other knee and stretching your other side. Your spine should feel long and even.

Hold Downward-Facing Dog Pose for fifteen to twenty seconds and then release, coming into Child's Pose to rest.

The more ease and comfort you find in a pose, the more your mind will be able to soften and relax. Try these two variations—even if you feel reasonably good in your Down Dog.

Variation 1: Supported Downward-Facing Dog Pose

There are a few ways to support your Downward-Facing Dog Pose. If your shoulders or wrists are uncomfortable with the pressure of the pose, start on all fours and place your hands on blocks. The blocks help you to lift through your shoulders and lengthen your spinal muscles more, alleviating some of the pressure in your wrists and shoulders, and you can get the feeling of your spinal muscles elongating, releasing tension. If your hands slip on the blocks, wrap the edge of a mat up around the blocks.

If your hamstrings and/or hips are very tight, and if placing your hands on blocks didn't relieve pressure in your wrists and shoulders, try Down Dog with your hands on the seat of a chair as shown in figure 4.7. Place a sturdy chair on your mat against a wall. Stand in front of the chair, place

YOGA FOR A HEALTHY LOWER BACK

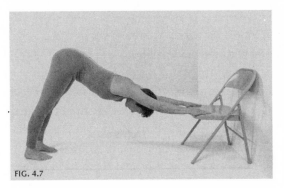
FIG. 4.7

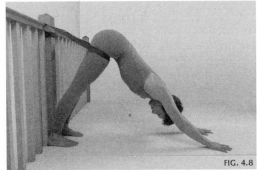
FIG. 4.8

your hands on the seat, and slowly walk your feet back until you feel a comfortable stretch in your trunk. You will probably feel a pretty good stretch in your hamstrings too—this is a good thing! As I mentioned in the beginning of this chapter, the tone of your hamstrings has a major effect on the health of your lower back. Bringing flexibility into your hamstrings and hips will help your lumbar muscles come into their natural alignment.

Variation 2: Dangling Down-Dog Pose

One of the best ways to release tightness in your lower back and balance your hips, sacral band, and the musculature along the sides of your spine is to practice Down Dog with the support of a belt around your hips. There are two ways to do it:

- Ask a friend to wrap a belt around the base of your hips and then gently draw evenly back on the sides of the belt.
- Wrapping a belt around any strong and stable support in your home (such as a support post in a basement or a sturdy banister) is worth trying, because it so effectively releases the gravitational pressure in your spine. Step into the belt. Lean your weight against it and bring your hands onto the floor or blocks. Walk your feet back until they are behind your hips, resting your heels up on a wall or banister posts if your heels do not reach the floor. Walk your blocks forward until you feel lightness in your hands and a release through your spinal muscles (fig. 4.8).

Deep Side Stretch Pose

Stretch and Strengthen | Parshvottanasana Variations

To set up for this pose, stand in the center of your mat and step your feet about four feet apart. Turn your left toes inward until they are at about a forty-five-degree angle to the right, and turn your right foot and leg ninety degrees to the right. Place a yoga block on either side of your right foot. Place your hands on your hips and turn your hips and torso to face your right foot. Balance your waist, chest, and shoulders evenly from left to right. Place one hand on your low abdomen and the other on your sacral joints. Drop your tailbone toward the floor and lift your front hip bones up toward your chest, bringing your hips into an upright and neutral position. This "neutral hip position" should be very familiar to you by now (for a refresher, see page 16).

Step 1: Half Deep Side Stretch Pose

With an inhalation, reach your arms over your head with your palms facing each other, and with an exhalation, bend your trunk forward over your right leg. The forward-bending action should come as much as possible from your hip joints, rather than from your middle or upper back. Reach your arms forward and then bring your hands to your blocks, or place your hands on the floor next to your right foot if your hamstrings are flexible. If your hamstrings are tight and it's difficult for you to reach the blocks while keeping your right leg straight, place your hands on the seat of a chair instead. Lift your trunk so it is parallel to the floor, with the front of your torso as long as possible (fig. 4.9). Draw your shoulder blades away from your neck and look forward, lengthening your breastbone and collarbones as much as possible.

Take a moment here to bring your hips into alignment with each other so your lower back can lengthen evenly on both sides. Place one hand on the back of your hips and adjust them so they are balanced. As in Half Forward Bend Pose (page 108), your back hips should be parallel to the floor so that your sacral joints are in

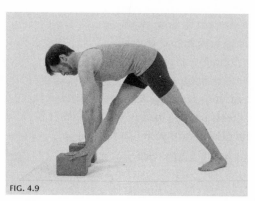

FIG. 4.9

YOGA FOR A HEALTHY LOWER BACK

natural alignment with your back hip bones. Stay here for a few breaths, feeling your lower back muscles lengthening as they get ready to come into a full forward bend. If you feel a strong stretch in your hamstrings, support your hands on more height. To come out of the pose, first place your hands on your hips, then lift your trunk back to an upright position. Rest for a few breaths. If your lower back feels comfortable, repeat the pose and move into the next step.

Step 2: Deep Side Stretch Pose

Start in step 1. On an exhalation, draw your spine down toward your right leg. Visualize that one day your trunk will come to rest on your right leg with your chin resting on your shin. If you are very flexible, you might experience this restful position today, but be sure your hips are balanced as you bend. In the final pose, all your back muscles, especially those of your lower back, get a good stretch, as do the hamstrings of your front leg, the calf of your back leg, and your hips.

To come out of the pose, first, lift your trunk so it is parallel with the floor. Take your hands on your hips, and with an inhalation, lift your trunk to an upright position. Turn your feet to the opposite direction, and repeat the pose to your left.

Deep Side Stretch Pose is excellent for lower back issues because the actions of moving into and out of the pose both lengthen and strengthen your lumbar muscles. As you bend forward and come into spinal flexion, you stretch and release tension all along your lower back. As you come up and out of the pose, you strengthen the musculature as you lift yourself up. If your back feels comfortable, you can flow into and out of the pose three or four times on each side, but caution is advised in the case of disk injuries, arthritis, spinal stenosis, or spondylolisthesis.

Variation: Open-Heart and Standing Seal

When you feel stable and comfortable in Deep Side Stretch Pose, try a more challenging variation that will increase tone in the stabilizing muscles of your legs, hips, and spine, as well as stretching the pectoralis minor muscles on your upper chest. You'll learn a lot more about the upper chest and upper back in chapter 6, but it's appropriate to note here that tightness in these muscles pulls the shoulder blades away from the centerline of the spine,

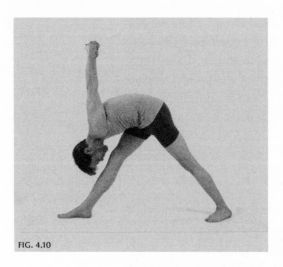

FIG. 4.10

which rounds the upper back and weakens its musculature. Toning them contributes to proper alignment of the shoulder blades and the tone of the upper back.

Standing in the starting position, interlace your hands behind your back. Stretch your shoulders back and reach your arms toward your back foot, mindfully lengthening your lumbar spine by scooping your tailbone in and up. Lift up your chest and look up toward the sky as you inhale. Open your heart!

Bend forward from your hips on your next exhalation. Descend your trunk toward your front leg as you lift your clasped hands up toward the ceiling (fig. 4.10). Feel the energy of your body drawing inward as you come into a forward bend; imagine you have sealed your physical and mental energy within yourself as you folded your trunk down toward your front leg. Hold the pose for a few breaths, then inhale, elongate your trunk forward, and come back to an upright position. Repeat to the opposite side.

Half-Moon Pose

Stretch and Strengthen | Ardha Chandrasana

Half-Moon Pose is one of the most beautiful standing poses, with therapeutic benefits including toning and strengthening all the main movers and supporters of your legs, hips, spine (especially your lower back), and shoulder girdle. In the pose, you'll feel your back leg sweeping upward from the earth just like the curved outline of a half moon, while your arms stretch away from each other so your inner light pours forth from your heart.

You can practice Half-Moon Pose with or without support for your body. Since balancing in Half-Moon Pose can be a challenge, practice it first with your back body supported at a wall. Slowly move away from the wall as you learn to balance on your own.

Begin with your back body two to three inches from a wall, and take your legs four to five feet apart. Turn your left foot slightly inward and turn your right leg all the way to the right, as you did for Triangle Pose on page 69. Place a block or chair against the wall, about a foot in front of your right toes.

Bend at your right hip and reach your trunk and right arm to the right, coming into Triangle Pose for a few moments. Feel your lower back elongating, and feel your hips as broad and open. Bend your right knee and place your right hand on your block or chair. Step your left foot to the right, sweep your left leg up, and stretch it straight. Feel your back body supported by the wall so you can stay in the pose for a few breaths without worrying about losing your balance (fig. 4.11).

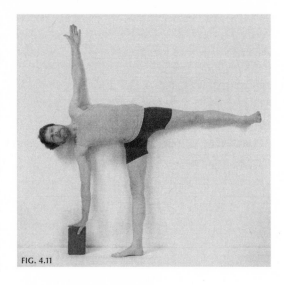

FIG. 4.11

Stretch your body from your left foot to the crown of your head, and from the tips of your right fingers to the tips of your left. Turn your torso up toward the sky any amount possible. Enjoy a feeling of openness in your hips, length in your spine, and a quiet, focused mind that brings you into a place of mental peace.

Flowing Bridge Pose

Strengthen | Setu Bandha Sarvangasana Variation

You learned Bridge Pose and its one-legged variation in chapter 2 as ways to stretch and strengthen your hips. Bridge Pose is a multibenefit pose, so now you'll practice a flowing version of it with the intention of strengthening your lower back muscles. Please review the basics about coming into Bridge Pose on page 56, and set your body up in the same way.

With an inhalation, lift your hips up as far as you comfortably can. Lift up your lower, middle, and upper back, and as you move, lift your arms all the way up over your head to the floor (fig. 4.12). As you exhale, slowly bring your spine down to the floor, vertebra by vertebra, at the same time that your arms come back down to your sides. Repeat four or five times, and coordinate the movements of your hips, trunk, arms, and breath, so your body feels like a smooth, undulating flow of energy from your feet up to your hands.

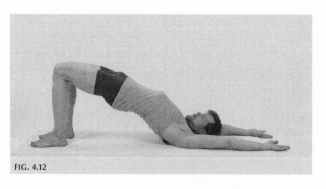

FIG. 4.12

The continuous movement of your spine into a backbend and then back down to the floor is very toning for the muscles in your lower back. If you have disk injuries, arthritis, or spinal stenosis, only lift your hips as high as your lumbar spine is comfortable. Over time you'll be able to lift up into a stronger backbend. Mindful movements are important here so that you don't overwork your shoulders, middle and upper back, or neck. Be sure to initiate your movements from the strength of your legs, your buttock muscles, and your abdominal core.

Flying Locust Pose

Strengthen | Shalabhasana Variation 1

This pose is a wonderful strengthener for your lower back muscles. Before you try it, though, be sure your sacrum feels comfortable in Alternate Arm/Leg Prone Backbend and Supported Locust Pose, both of which you practiced in chapter 3 (pages 105 and 106). Also, now would be a good time to review "Tips for Healthy Backbends" (page 103).

When you're ready to practice Flying Locust Pose, lie on your front body and place your hands under your thighs, palms up. Pressing your hips down into your hands so your tailbone is moving toward the floor, raise both legs upward as you inhale, stretching them straight. Bring them down to rest as you exhale; repeat two more times and rest for a few breaths with your forehead on your hands.

Now stretch your arms forward, press your hips and legs strongly down, and lift your arms, shoulders, and head up with an inhalation. Bring them down to rest as you exhale and relax again with your forehead on your hands. If either of these actions is difficult for you, practice them individually until you feel ready to proceed into full Flying Locust Pose. When you can easily lift your legs and arms, you are ready to proceed.

For full Flying Locust Pose, lie stretched straight on your front body, with your arms and legs straight and engaged. Draw your shoulder blades away from your neck. With an inhalation, lift your arms, shoulders, head, and legs (fig. 4.13). Look forward, or look down at the floor if your neck feels compressed. Keep your legs straight with your toes pointing straight back.

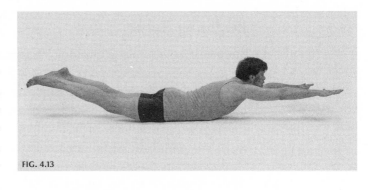

FIG. 4.13

Turn your palms toward each other to ease any pressure in your shoulder joints. Hold the pose for about ten seconds, then release and rest.

Flying Locust Pose is a true test of sacral and lower back tone, and any time you spend in it or working up to it is "money in the lower-back bank." When you strengthen and tone the musculature of your back, along with toning your abdominal core, as you will in chapter 5, your body will become self-supporting.

Swimming Locust Pose

Strengthen | Shalabhasana Variation 2

Once you can hold Flying Locust, you can go swimming! Start in full Flying Locust Pose. As you inhale, spread your arms and legs wide apart from each other and bring them back together as you exhale. Repeat these movements a number of times—aim to continue your flow for six or seven breaths. Besides being a fun movement to coordinate in your body, Swimming Locust Pose is an excellent way to strengthen your hips and lower back.

Note that both Flying Locust and Swimming Locust Poses can be deeply challenging for anyone with a tight and restricted sacrum. If you can't do these poses, or if you can only do them for a moment or two, don't despair or heap judgment on yourself. Remember, you are on a journey toward lower back health, and having goals like Swimming Locust Pose can keep you motivated to continue to balance and strengthen your lower back.

Reclining Bolster Twist

Stretch | Jathara Parivartanasana Variation 1

This supported reclining twist gently massages your sacral joints and lower back, where you have just done a lot of work in Flying and Swimming Locust Poses. You can start slowly, taking your knees down partway at first to make sure your back is comfortable, and increase the twist as you progress. For less stretch, place a block in the "high" position against each side of the bolster to support your thighs.

Lie on your back with your feet flat on the floor and with a bolster by your side. Lift your hips and slide the bolster underneath them. The bolster should completely support your hips; the top edge of the bolster should touch your lower back ribs. Hold the sides of the bolster with your hands. Press your shoulders down toward the floor and lift your front ribs, creating length and space in your abdomen and chest as if you were practicing Bridge Pose. Draw your right knee toward your chest, then your left knee. Your thighs should be perpendicular to the floor, knees pointing straight up. Take your arms straight out to the sides.

Take a long, deep inhalation, feeling your chest expand with the infusion of prana, and as you exhale, take your legs down to the right until your right thigh rests on the bolster or on your block (fig. 4.14). With an inhalation lift them back up to center, and exhale them down to your left, resting your left thigh on the bolster. If you feel too much challenge bringing your legs back up, draw your knees toward your armpit first and then lift your legs, or lift your legs one at a time. Mindfully move your legs in sync with the rhythm of your breath—Ocean Breath (see page 12) is excellent for this kind of gentle movement. Visualize your sacral joints lengthening and your lower back releasing tension, and feel that your spinal muscles are massaged by the twisting action of your legs. If you have a misalignment in your sacral joints, pay careful attention to each side; if one side feels achy, do not practice the pose to that side until you've created more stability in the joints.

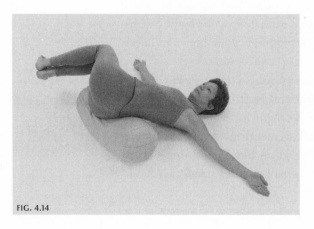

FIG. 4.14

Inverted Cleanser Pose

Rest | Viparita Karani Variations

I'll show two ways to practice Inverted Cleanser Pose. One is a freestanding version that requires a little action through your legs, bringing a refreshing feeling of stimulation and newly circulated prana through your body. The other is a restorative version with your body completely supported by props, sometimes known, for obvious reasons, as Legs-Up-the-Wall Pose. It's good to practice this version when you are ready to completely rest and relax. You can practice both and use them as your body requests. Many students tell me that they prefer the freestanding version, because their legs don't fall asleep.

Inverted Cleanser Pose rests the back in a gentle backbend. It is called *Viparita Karani* in Sanskrit, which is often translated as "reverse process." When the body is in an upside-down position—with the legs and hips above the head—blood flows with gravity from the feet down into the heart. The heart can then rest, because blood is flowing fully and easily into the brain. Gravity also helps lymphatic fluids flow into the endocrine glands in the torso, throat, and head. The gentle back-bending action of the pose massages and stimulates the kidneys and adrenals, which we've learned are crucial components of lower back health.

Hold either variation of Inverted Cleanser Pose for a few minutes at least, and hold Restorative Cleanser for five or ten minutes so your body can reap the benefits of physically relaxing and becoming energetically restored and renewed. Women, during your menstrual cycle, please practice Inverted Cleanser Pose with your hips flat on the floor.

Variation 1: Active Cleanser

Come into this variation right after you've practiced Reclining Bolster Twist. From the twist, bring your legs back to the center and, leaving your bolster under your hips, lift your legs, one at a time, up toward the ceiling, as straight as you can (fig. 4.15). Check that your abdomen is long and soft and your chest is open. If your hamstrings are tight or if you get tired, bend your knees and let your feet hang toward the floor while your thighs stay upright for a moment. You can adjust the height under your hips until your back is very comfortable. Many students are surprised that a folded blanket (or even another bolster) on top of the first bolster creates freedom in the chest and abdomen.

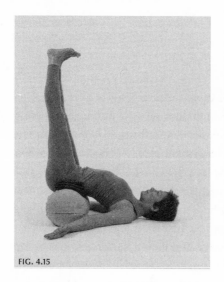

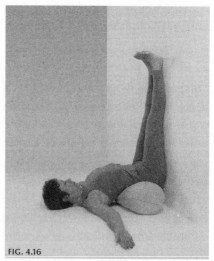

FIG. 4.15

FIG. 4.16

To come out of Active Cleanser, bend your knees one at a time back into your chest, and place your feet on the floor one at a time. Lift your hips up and slide your bolster and/or blankets out. Lie with your back flat on the floor and hug your knees to your chest to gently massage your lower back.

Variation 2: Restorative Cleanser

Lie on your back with your legs vertically up a wall and a bolster, folded blanket, or block nearby. Place your hips and back thighs as close to the wall as possible. Bend your knees and press the soles of your feet into the wall. Lift your hips and place your bolster, blanket, or block horizontally under your hips. Your abdomen should be horizontal and your navel should gently sink down toward your spine (fig. 4.16). You can adjust the height under your hips, adding more or taking some away until your back is very comfortable. Press your shoulders down and open your heart to create a slight backbend in your upper chest; maintain the lift in your chest as you relax your shoulders. If you can't rest your thighs on the wall, place a bolster upright behind them. For even more relaxation in your legs, belt your thighs or shins together and let your legs rest into the pressure of the belt.

To come out of Restorative Cleanser, bend your knees and slowly roll over onto one side of your body. Lie flat on the floor and draw your knees to your chest to gently massage your lower back.

Deep Relaxation: Experience Your Body's Softness

Rest | Shavasana Variation 3

This resting position facilitates the release of your lower back while it is in a supported position. It's a good choice for practicing deep relaxation after you've worked to stretch and strengthen your lower back. Remember to ask your mind to stay present, quiet, and focused on your lower back so you notice how your yoga practice has opened, softened, and strengthened it.

Lie down on the floor or on a blanket with your lower legs and heels resting on the seat of a chair. Choose a chair that supports your calves at a height where your thighs feel as though they were pouring easily from the chair into your hips. Your lower back should be comfortable (if it isn't, try placing a rolled towel at any point underneath it) and it should feel quiet and gently elongated. Support your neck and head with a rolled, folded blanket so that it, too, is long and comfortable (fig. 4.17). For a soothing feeling in your belly and lower back, lay a folded blanket across your abdomen for gentle but supportive pressure.

Feel your legs, hips, and lower back deeply relaxing. Breathe into your spine. As you inhale, visualize your spine elongating from your hips to the back of your head, and as you exhale, let your body completely rest and be held by the earth. Let your neck rest deeply into its support and visualize all the neck, upper back, and middle back muscles letting go.

Now focus your awareness on where your sacral and lumbar spines meet, at that precious joint between the L5 and S1 vertebrae. Visualize the natural, slightly upward curve of L5 and S1. Visualize the disk between L5 and S1 as soft and spongy, filled with resiliency. As you slowly and mindfully inhale, mentally travel up through each lumbar vertebra from L5 to L1, visualizing each disk with the same qualities; soft, spongy, and elastic. Each time you slowly and mindfully exhale, visualize all the muscles around your lower back draping down and resting along the floor. Let your lower back breathe and relax.

Observe how your intention to practice yoga for the health and happiness of your lower back has made a change there. Perhaps it is giving you less "feedback," which means

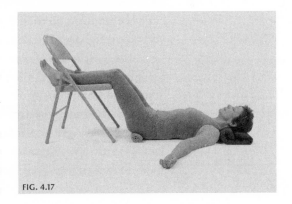

FIG. 4.17

it's more comfortable because you have massaged and toned your muscles, allowing blood and spinal fluid to flow smoothly through your spine. In a holistic view, your practice has also had an effect on the kidneys and adrenals, affording them the room they need to physically function, and, energetically, to modulate the fight-or-flight response in balance with the relaxation response. Visualize prana flowing around your lower back through the Ida and Pingala, the left and right energy channels along your spine. Visualize how the energy of the Ida and Pingala nadis meet at your Manipura chakra, right behind your navel, and how prana flows all around your navel, through your abdomen, and back into your lower back. Feel your lower back massaged by yoga poses, nourished by the flow of energy, and resting in balance.

Grow and Progress

Marichi's Seated Twist

Stretch | Marichyasana I

This is a soothing twist that provides a stable position for your sacrum while it stretches all the lower back myofascia and massages your kidneys and your adrenal glands. Practice the final stage only when your lower back is comfortable with spinal twists.

Sit on the floor with your legs straight in front of you. If this is difficult, sit on a folded blanket. Bend your right knee and place your right foot on the floor inside your left thigh, but not quite touching it. Your foot should be in line with your right sit bone. Be sure your right and left buttocks are equally grounded into the earth or your blanket. Lean back, place both hands behind you on the floor, and arch your back up toward the ceiling as you take a big, deep inhalation.

Lift your chest any amount possible. Imagine your chest as a beautiful fountain of energy and light. Now, maintaining the lifting feeling through your chest, bring your spine back to an upright position. With your next inhalation, lift your right arm up. Deeply exhale while you turn to your left and bring your right arm to the inside of your right leg. Your right inner leg should gently press against your right arm in order to keep your right thigh and shin in an upright position. Fold your right arm at your elbow and raise your hand so your palm faces outward. Keep your left hand on the floor behind you (fig. 4.18).

With each inhalation, elongate your spine upward, from the base of your hips to the crown of your head. Energetically, you can encourage the lift of your trunk and feel great support for your spine by coming into Root Lock, or Mula Bandha, which I introduced on page 39. As you inhale, feel energy lifting through your trunk and broadening your upper chest. With each exhalation, deepen the twist by turning your trunk farther to the left. Go mindfully and slowly, feeling how the twist speaks to your spine. Use the connection between your left arm and right thigh to help turn your torso more. Finally, turn your head to the left and gaze over your left shoulder.

If your spine is happy, try moving into the final stage of the pose: Exhaling, wrap your right arm around your right shin, reach your left arm behind your back, and clasp your hands together. If you can't quite connect your hands, hold a belt between your hands. Remember to breathe fully in this deep twist.

There are many benefits to seated twists. They are helpful in releasing tightness in the spinal muscles and lengthening the entire spine, helping the vertebrae to shift into proper alignment. They create gentle traction in the spine, especially the lower back. In the case of disk injuries, the traction can create height at the intervertebral spaces, which brings elasticity into

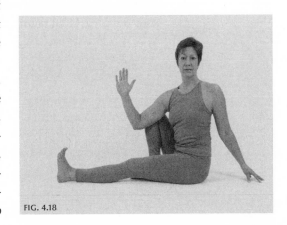

FIG. 4.18

the disks and can help relieve pain. Finally, twists massage the inner organs and help the endocrine system to come into balance. You can see why this pose is a great way to expand your yoga practice for lower back health!

A word of caution is appropriate for those with a herniated disk condition, though. Approach Marichi's Seated Twist slowly, moving just a little at a time into the pose. Listen to the feedback in your lower back and be sure it's comfortable before you progress into a deep twist.

Revolved Wide-Legged Seated Pose

Stretch | Parivrtta Upavishta Konasana

Sit again, with your hips on the floor and your legs straight forward. Now take your legs out to the sides so your feet are about four feet apart. You are now in Wide-Legged Seated Pose. Take a minute to do a self-assessment of your hips and spine. Place one hand on the back of your hips and the other on your lower abdomen. Bring your hips into neutral position. Both front and back hips should be lifting upright, with a slight inward curvature of your lumbar spine. Your abdominal wall should be active and engaged to help support your lower back. If this isn't how your body feels, place a folded blanket under your hips; this will help you to sit upright. Place your hands lightly on the floor behind you, and lift your trunk up toward the ceiling while you simultaneously press your thighs down into the earth.

With an inhalation, walk your right hand over to the inside of your right knee, and as you exhale, stretch the right side of your torso toward your right leg. Hold your right big toe with your right hand. Your right arm

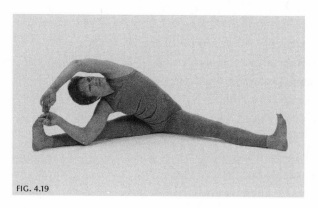

FIG. 4.19

should touch your inner right leg. If you can't reach your foot, wrap a belt around your foot and hold the belt. You can also bend your right knee to ease tightness in your right adductor (inner thigh) and hamstring muscles.

Place your left hand on your left thigh and with an exhalation, turn your torso up toward the ceiling. Your torso, shoulders, and head should be in line with your right leg. Gaze to your left; as you turn your torso upward and if your neck is agreeable, turn your head and look toward the sky.

Have a dialogue with your lower back before you proceed to the final pose. Ask it how it's feeling and listen carefully—it will tell you everything you need to know. As your lower back releases into the stretch, move with your exhalations, drawing your trunk closer to your right leg and deepening the stretch by turning more and more.

Finally, lift your left arm up and reach it over your left ear. If your lower back is very flexible, hold your right foot with your left hand (fig. 4.19). Feel your hips and legs well grounded, and enjoy the feeling of your spine becoming light and open.

This pose stretches and tones the quadratus lumborum muscles, as well as the erector spinae group and the latissimus dorsi muscles, which are often indicated in lower back pain. Stretching away from the side of your back that feels tight and painful can bring significant relief. If you have an active and painful lower back or sacral injury, go only as far as your body is quite comfortable. Come out of the pose with a deep inhalation, then repeat it to the other side.

Balanced Warrior Pose

Stretch and Strengthen | Virabhadrasana III

Now that you've stretched and toned your lower back, you're ready to try Balanced Warrior Pose, also known as "Warrior III." This pose is challenging, requiring flexibility in your hamstrings, hips, chest, and shoulders, so we'll begin by practicing Half Balanced Warrior Pose, where you'll strengthen your lower back as you work on finding your balance on one leg. Balanced Warrior is a strong pose, and you can use Ocean Breath to help support yourself and keep your energy concentrated and even. Once you do, you'll find a sense of empowerment and inner strength; your inner warrior will be awakened!

Step 1: Half Balanced Warrior Pose

Stand in Mountain Pose with your feet grounded, and sense the energy of the earth lifting up from the soles of your feet to the crown of your head.

Feel yourself tall and strong. Exhaling, come into Standing Forward Bend Pose (page 109). Lift your head and shoulders up and look forward, making your trunk as long as possible. If your hands don't reach the floor, place them on blocks. Shift your weight onto your right foot and with an exhalation, lift your left leg straight back and up until it is parallel to the floor (fig. 4.20). Stretch your left leg strongly and make your body as long as possible from your left foot to the crown of your head.

Take a moment to gauge how much support is appropriate for your body. If your hamstrings feel uncomfortably stretched or if you can't straighten your right knee, place your hands on a chair instead of on blocks. Hold the pose for ten seconds, and bring your left foot back down to the floor. Come out of Standing Forward Bend and take a break, then repeat the pose lifting your right leg up.

Step 2: Full Balanced Warrior Pose

Stand in Mountain Pose and shift your weight onto your right foot. With an inhalation lift your arms over your head, palms facing each other. You are now in Upward Hand Pose. On an exhalation, bend forward from your hips. Reach your trunk and arms strongly forward as you bring them half-way down to the floor. At the same time that your trunk is descending, lift your left leg up and back the way you did in Half Balanced Warrior Pose.

Your trunk, arms, and left leg should be a straight, powerful line, per-pendicular to your grounded right leg. Be sure your head is aligned with your spine—your ears should be in line with your arms. Gaze at the floor until you feel balanced, then look forward (fig. 4.21).

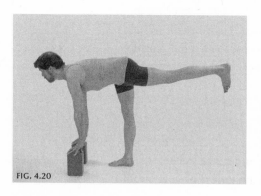

FIG. 4.20

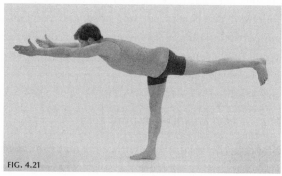

FIG. 4.21

YOGA FOR A HEALTHY LOWER BACK

Keep your right leg strong, and balance on your right foot for a few breaths. Hold the pose for ten to fifteen seconds if possible. Stretch your left leg back while your spine stretches forward, all the way through the crown of your head and the tips of your fingers. Lift your abdominal wall slightly up toward your spine to engage your abdominal core and balance the pose from your center. To come out of the pose, simply retrace your steps, bringing your left foot to the floor as your trunk and arms lift up, coming back into Upward Hand Pose. Take a couple of breaths, arms still raised, and repeat Balanced Warrior Pose to the opposite side.

Variation: Proud Warrior Flow

Once you feel comfortable moving into and out of Balanced Warrior from Upward Hand Pose, you can challenge yourself to come into it from Proud Warrior Pose, which you practiced on page 119.

Come into Proud Warrior with your right leg forward and your left leg back. On an exhalation, fold forward, bringing your trunk and arms parallel to the floor. Lengthen your trunk forward any amount possible. On your next inhalation step your left foot toward your right foot and lift your left leg up and back until it is parallel to the floor. Straighten your right leg as you lift your left leg. Hold Balanced Warrior for ten to fifteen seconds, focusing your mind on finding its balance, strength, and inner poise.

To come out of this variation, first come back into Proud Warrior: Bend your right knee, reach your left leg back and place your left foot on the floor while you lift your trunk and arms back up. Inhale as you straighten your right leg. Turn your feet so they are parallel to each other and then repeat the pose to your left.

Cobra Pose Flow

Strengthen | Bhujangasana Variations

Before you practice Cobra Pose, take a moment to review "Tips for Healthy Backbends" on page 103 and make sure your lower back is comfortable practicing Supported Cobra Pose (page 104). When it is, you're ready to move into full Cobra Pose. The intention of Cobra Pose is to strengthen the musculature of your lower back without causing your spinal muscles to contract too much, which would put you at risk for muscle spasms and injury. Be sure to mindfully observe your body as you practice each step, and only proceed as far as your body says it's ready to go.

Step 1: Sphinx Pose

Lie down on your front body, resting your head either on your forehead or chin, whichever is most comfortable for your head and neck. Place your hands on the floor forward of your shoulders, and draw your arms next to the sides of your body, with your forearms on the floor and your elbows by your ribs. Spread your fingers and ground your palms. Slowly lift your head and shoulders up while your hips and legs press firmly down into the ground. Engage your buttocks. Roll your shoulders back and draw them away from your ears, so your collarbones are high and your heart is open and broad. Look forward and elongate the back of your head. Draw your chest away from your waist as you lift it up, creating length and traction along your spine (fig. 4.22). Hold for ten to fifteen seconds while you listen to the feedback from your lower back. Come down and rest. If your lower back is comfortable, proceed to Cobra-in-the-Grass Pose. Otherwise, repeat Sphinx Pose.

Step 2: Cobra-in-the-Grass Pose

Now you'll begin the transition into Full Cobra. Start in Sphinx Pose, but this time place your hands by your shoulders and lift your forearms and elbows off the floor. Keeping your elbows bent, gently draw the right side of your torso forward, then the left side. Slide from left to right, creating a gentle swaying, slightly twisting action from side to side, elongating your spine forward and lifting it upward little by little (fig. 4.23). Visualize a snake in the grass. If you've ever watched a snake move through grass, you

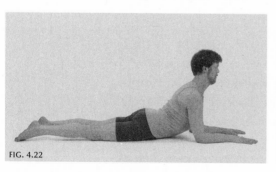
FIG. 4.22

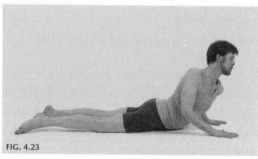
FIG. 4.23

YOGA FOR A HEALTHY LOWER BACK

know how intuitive and Zen-like its movements are—it smoothly glides around obstacles, lifting its head to see what's ahead, then sinking it back down as it proceeds with determination and stealth. Bring that same strong, focused intention to your practice of this pose.

Step 3: Full Cobra Pose

After your curvy grass-traveling Cobra has warmed your lower back muscles, you're ready for the full pose. Start as you did in step 2, and, pressing your hands down, lift your trunk and slowly straighten your arms, using them to lift your spine into more and more of a backbend. Practice all the actions of step 1 and engage your abdominal core muscles, to make sure you are supporting your lower back.

Stretch your arms only as straight as your lower back comfortably allows—it's absolutely fine to keep your elbows bent so your back can benefit from a healthy, but not overdone, stretch (fig. 4.24). Your lower back muscles should feel engaged but not compressed or gripping. Your legs and front groins should remain well grounded on the floor. If it's comfortable in your neck, take your head back, but keep your gaze soft and focused inward. And if your lower back gives you full permission, straighten your arms fully and come into the strongest version of the pose.

Visualize each spinal vertebra, from S1 all the way through your lower, middle, and upper back, lifting up and coming into a gentle, even back arch, a luminous strand of pearls connected and energized by the flow of prana through the Sushumna, the central energy channel of your spine.

To come out of Cobra Pose, slowly bring your spine down to the ground, vertebra by vertebra. Place your forearms parallel to the top of your mat and briefly rest your forehead on your hands. Then place your left hand flat on the floor, roll over onto the right side of your body, and come up to a seated position. After a strong backbend such as Cobra Pose it feels great to release your lower back, first by lengthening it, then by resting it in a completely supported position. I recommend that you practice Forward-Bending Hero's Pose, (page 107) for a few moments to stretch your spine, and then come into Decompressing Standing Forward Bend (page 110), placing a

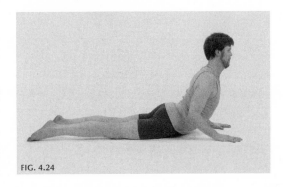

FIG. 4.24

rolled blanket between your thighs and abdomen. Breathe deeply into your lower back, feeling it rest into the blanket support—softening, releasing, undoing.

Head-to-Knee Pose

Stretch | Janu Shirshasana

Sit on your mat with your legs straight forward, and have a belt handy. Bend your left knee and bring your left foot to rest along your inner upper right thigh. Be sure you are sitting squarely on your sit bones. Place your hands on your lower back and feel that your hips and lower back are lifting up and you are in neutral hip position. Lift your arms and trunk up, as if coming into Upward Hand Pose, then fold forward at your hips and hold your right foot with your hands. If you can't reach your foot or if your lower back is uncomfortable, hold your foot with a belt (fig. 4.25). Keep your trunk upright and breathe deeply for a few moments.

Turn your trunk to align your spine with your right leg. Exhaling, fold more deeply from your hips and reach forward through your trunk (fig. 4.26). *Forward* is the important direction of movement, so that your whole trunk elongates, rather than overrounds in your lower or middle back.

A forward bend should be a comfortable stretch for your lower back; it requires length all along the back body, from your calf, into your hamstrings, through your hips, and all along your spine. If there's discomfort

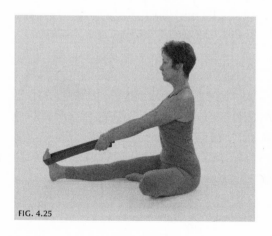

FIG. 4.25

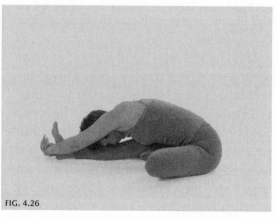

FIG. 4.26

YOGA FOR A HEALTHY LOWER BACK

anywhere along the back of your body, keep your trunk lifting upward; you can also keep your right knee bent. As your hamstrings, hips, and spinal muscles lengthen over time, you'll be able to stretch your spine forward and straighten your leg, moving more deeply into the wonderful feeling of quiet repose that forward bends offer.

Stay in the pose for fifteen to twenty seconds, using the ebb and flow of your breath to reach your trunk farther toward your foot as you inhale, and gently releasing it down toward your right thigh as you exhale. Finally, gaze down at your thigh while you maintain a comfortable position for your neck. When you're ready to come out, lift your trunk halfway up, stretch your arms and trunk back up to a seated Upward Hand Pose, and then release your arms down. Change legs and repeat with your right leg bent.

Seated Forward Bend Pose

Stretch | Paschimottanasana

Sit in Staff Pose and check that you are in neutral hip position. If your lower back is rounding or collapsing back, sit on a folded blanket. Have a belt nearby. Inhaling, reach your arms and trunk up and with a deep exhalation, reach forward, just as you did in Head-to-Knee Pose, and hold your feet (fig. 4.27). If you can't reach, hold your feet with a belt. Also, as in Head-to-Knee

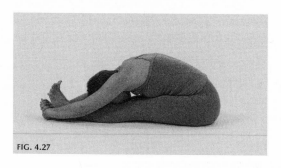

FIG. 4.27

Pose, you can bend your knees to learn how to fold forward with your trunk long.

Inhaling, lift your trunk slightly and look forward. Exhaling, move more deeply into a forward bend as your hamstrings, hips, and spinal muscles release. As you gaze toward your legs, don't let your head or neck be "pushy"; by that I mean don't let them try to push your trunk into the pose. Repeat this process of mindfully moving for a few breaths, each breath offering an opportunity for your physical body to release into the pose and for your mind and emotions to come into a place of quiet and repose.

Stay in the pose for fifteen to twenty seconds, or longer if you are comfortable. When you are ready to come out, look forward and lift your spine halfway up, then reach your trunk and arms upward into a seated Upward Hand Pose before you release them to the floor.

Before you rest in a well-earned Child's Pose, check in with your lower back. If it feels tired from forward bending, lie down on your back and come into a very gentle Bridge Pose (page 56) for ten seconds or so to return your lower back to its natural alignment, then hug your knees into your chest.

Child's Pose and Deep Relaxation

Rest | Balasana and Shavasana Variation 3

Child's Pose is a great "go-to" pose at the end of any practice, especially when you've worked hard to strengthen, lengthen, and tone your back. And you've done just that! Rest now in Child's Pose (page 61) for a few moments to completely relax your lower back. Visualize your lumbar spine once again as a luminous pearl necklace, now in a gentle upward curve supported by the flow of breath into your abdomen and lower back. Visualize each end of your lumbar spine gently floating down into a subtle upside-down U, one end meeting your sacral spine and the other meeting your thoracic spine. With each inhalation, visualize your breath as the necklace's threads, gently elongating and spreading the pearls apart from each other, and enjoy a feeling of spaciousness in your lower back. With each exhalation, let the threads of the necklace soften and relax, releasing the pearls down so you can rest in the support of toned muscles and the flow of vital prana.

You may wish to continue to rest in the Shavasana we practiced on page 157.

5

Your Abdominal Core

How often do you think about your midsection? Your tummy? Your gut? Your "six-pack"? Your "twelve-pack"? I'm going to guess you spend a few hours each day focused on it without even realizing it.

If you are conscious of your body image, you probably think about your belly first thing in the morning and last thing at night—looking at it, judging it, letting it set your mood, and choosing your clothes for the day based on how flat, round, small, or big you think it is. Like with your lower back, you may also have invested in products marketed as quick fixes for your abs.

Your stomach is a highly communicative place in your body, in addition to being the source of body-image insecurity or pride. It prompts you to sit down to eat when you are hungry. It makes itself heard after you eat as well, either with pleasure when it feels full or with regret when you've eaten too much. If you are stressed out or tend toward anxiety, you may be hearing your stomach's call more—or less—often than usual, or you may find yourself addressing stomach acid issues an hour after every meal.

Let's face it—we are a stomach-obsessed culture, judging ourselves and others based on whether we can pinch more than an inch or have six-pack abs. Regardless of where on that spectrum you fall, it's likely you have a complicated relationship with your midsection.

The ancient yogis and other ancient cultures, though, understood the tremendous power that resides in the abdomen. They celebrated it as a source of creation, sensuality, and self-sustaining heat and energy from which we power ourselves throughout our lives.

You'll be happy to know that especially when seen through the yogic lens, you don't need six-pack abs to have excellent abdominal tone that supports and empowers the rest of your body. (Incidentally, on the topic of six-pack abs—though popular, the practice of "ab crunches" is not a favorite with me because crunches can irritate a sensitive lower back and overtighten psoas muscles. So there's no need to worry—we won't be doing any crunches in this book.)

The title of this chapter is "Your Abdominal Core," and I want you to take a moment to contemplate the notion of "core" before we dive in. Everything in your body, remember, is connected. Our work so far has painted a picture of the layers of wellness we're pursuing with our yoga practice: whole health starts with back health; back health starts with sacral health; sacral health requires hip and lumbar health. Now we come to the "core" from which all those other areas draw their strength—or recruit their weakness.

The core of an apple or pear contains its seeds, its hope for a healthy, "fruitful" future. So too is your abdominal core your innermost wellspring of strength, support, and wellness. Let's explore it together.

THROUGH WESTERN EYES: THE PHYSICAL VIEW

Your abdominal cavity is the largest cavity in your body. It includes the entire area from your pelvic floor muscles up to your diaphragm, encompassing the front, sides, and back of your middle body. It contains most of your internal organs, including the liver, spleen, pancreas, gall bladder, stomach, and intestines. Your abdomen isn't a mover or a shaker (well, sometimes it *does* shake . . .) the way your arms, legs, and spine are, but it affects and is affected by how you engage the rest of your body with movements and posture alike. A toned and engaged abdominal core has plenty of room to hold your internal organs without compressing or stressing them. Very importantly for our purposes, a healthy abdominal core will also contribute to the stability and fluidity of your lower back.

Your abdominal wall consists of four layers of muscles: the rectus abdominis, or the large muscles that run up the front of the abdomen; and the three layers of flat muscles that wrap around the abdomen. These "wrapping" muscles are the external obliques, internal obliques, and transversus abdominis muscles. More on each of those in a moment.

Together, the abdominal muscles act like flexible, woven layers of mesh that support your abdominal organs and lower back. They rotate your torso, help you bend forward and to the sides, and then they help you come back to an upright position. Toned abdominal muscles help protect your lumbar disks by supporting and stabilizing the movements of your spine. They also help you breathe, if you imagine a healthy breath as a three-dimensional action in which the rib cage expands forward, backward, and to the sides while the diaphragm rises and lowers into the abdominal cavity.[1]

The term *abdominal core* is now commonplace in the yoga world, not to mention in the fitness and athletic industries. Each discipline has its own interpretation of what makes up your "core." Sometimes just the innermost layers of abdominal and back muscles are included. Other definitions include the deep hip muscles, and other definitions go further to include the shoulders, hips, and legs. Since our main intention is to create a healthy lower back, we will focus on toning and balancing the musculature that directly affects the sacral and lumbar spines. So when I talk about the "abdominal core," I'm including your abdominals as described above, plus your psoas muscles, which you explored in chapters 2 and 3, and the muscles of the lower back, which you explored in chapter 4. These three areas are intricately connected—if the abdominals are weak and the psoas muscles are short, tight, or stronger than the abdominals, your lumbar spine will be pulled forward, straining the lower back and creating a lordosis (excess inward curvature of the lumbar spine). The lordosis in turn will tip your back hip bones forward, causing your lumbar muscles to shorten and tighten up, limiting your lower back's range of motion.

To avoid this dysfunction, this chapter focuses on toning and balancing your abdominal muscles so your abdominals, psoas, and lower back muscles work together with tone and balance. Then your abdominal core can support you and provide you with the mobility and flexibility you need to move through every day with ease and comfort.

Anatomy Lesson: Your Abdominal Muscles

As you continue on your journey toward a healthy lower back, it's worth taking the time to understand the basics of your abdominal muscles and how they help you in your daily life (illustration 16).

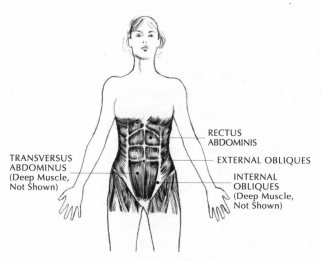

RECTUS
ABDOMINIS

EXTERNAL OBLIQUES

INTERNAL
OBLIQUES
(Deep Muscle,
Not Shown)

TRANSVERSUS
ABDOMINUS
(Deep Muscle,
Not Shown)

Illustration 16. The Muscles of the Abdominal Core

Let's start with the rectus abdominis, the outermost layer and the most prominent abdominal muscles. These muscles originate at the pubic bone and run along both sides of the linea alba, the flat band of connective tissue that runs along the center of your abdomen from your pubic bone to your breastbone. These are the muscles that are commonly called the "six-pack" because they are segmented into sections that become visible when the muscles are highly developed. The rectus abdominis help the spine and torso bend forward, and they stabilize your hips when you walk. Along with your psoas, they also control the tilt of your pelvic girdle, which is one reason these muscles are so important for your healthy lower back.

Next let's talk about the obliques. You have two sets of these important muscles. The external obliques are the large, broad muscles that run diagonally down and in from between your upper and middle ribs to the rim of your hip bones and the bottom of your linea alba. The internal obliques lie underneath the external obliques. They begin in the myofascia of the lower back and run up toward the midline of your body, to the upper ribs and the top of your linea alba. The obliques' primary function is in the rotation and side bending of your trunk. Toned internal and external oblique muscles support the lumbar spine during a twist, especially in that important spot between L5 and S1 where the disk is thicker and carries the weight and energy of a lot of movement. As I've said before, strong, healthy obliques maintain healthy pressure on the curve of the lower back, which helps to counteract any tendency of the lumbar spine to go into lordosis.

The deepest layer of muscles is the transversus abdominis. This set of muscles wraps horizontally all the way around your abdomen, starting at the lumbar and thoracic myofascia, passing over the lower ribs and iliac crest, and attaching to the linea alba and pubic bone in front. The transversus abdominis are often overlooked in conversations about your abdominal core because they aren't involved in the movement of your torso. But they are crucially important to your journey into wellness, as they act like a belt that supports the contents of your abdominal cavity.

The Brain-Gut Connection: The Vagus Nerve

Let's step back from muscles for a moment and discuss how your nervous system works in your abdominal core. One might call this the "brain-gut connection." The most important channel of communication between your brain and the internal organs, including those in your abdominal core, is the vagus nerve. Not to be indelicate, but if you have ever gotten a stomach bug and felt your heart pounding, sweat pouring, and mind racing—even to the point of passing out—you are intimately familiar with how powerful the vagus nerve is when it's "upset." At its best, though, the vagus nerve is an important pathway of relaxation and calm in your body. Yoga practice has a direct effect on the vagus nerve, so understanding it is valuable as we begin to work on your core.

The vagus nerve begins at the base of your brain and runs through your thoracic and abdominal cavities. It connects to and exerts control over most of your internal organs. In addition to conveying electrical impulses to your internal organs, it communicates information about the condition of your organs to your central nervous system. You may remember when I talked about the parasympathetic nervous system (PNS) back in chapter 1 (page 7). As part of its role as a liaison between your brain and organs, the vagus nerve controls parasympathetic stimulation of your heart, which can lead to a reduction in heart rate and blood pressure and creates a relaxation response throughout your body.[2]

Because your vagus nerve is so directly connected to your abdominal organs, including the stomach, kidneys, intestines, and liver, and because yoga directly stimulates the vagus nerve, your abdominal area is affected by every yoga pose I can think of. Standing poses and backbends stretch and elongate your abdominal organs; forward bends, twists, and abdominal poses massage them, and inversions relax gravitational forces on them. As your organs are stimulated by yoga poses, so is your vagus nerve and your parasympathetic nervous system.[3]

Your nervous system's relationship with your core body is also directly affected by pranayama, yogic breath practice. Three-Part Breath (page 41) brings deep inhalations into your pelvis, abdomen, and chest to release muscle tightness, and it encourages the vagus nerve to send your heart relaxing messages through your long, deep exhalations. In Ocean Breath (page 12), slow, elongated inhalations and exhalations enhance PNS activity and increase indicators of healthy vagus nerve function.[4] When you make your exhalations longer than your inhalations in Ocean Breath, you directly stimulate the PNS and elicit the relaxation response.[5]

The end result of pranayama practice is that your heart rate slows, your blood pressure drops, and you can move into a state of physical and mental calmness that can help you cope with, among other things, lower back pain.[6] But this deep sense of relaxation doesn't end on your yoga mat. Remember that you carry some of the calming effects of your practice into your daily life. With a relaxation response in your back pocket, you can be more present to all that goes on in your life—especially challenging situations— and face them with a resiliency that helps you maintain calm, balance, and equanimity.

In this chapter you'll practice yoga poses that tone your abdominal wall, massage your internal organs, and stimulate the parasympathetic nervous system through the vagus nerve. By the end of the chapter, your abdomen should feel alive and toned, and I hope your mind will feel calm and relaxed!

THROUGH EASTERN EYES: THE ENERGETIC VIEW

Have you ever heard of a yogi contemplating his navel? You may have heard the phrase as the punch line of a joke, but the practice actually has legitimate spiritual roots. I've talked about the third chakra—Manipura—which encompasses the area between your navel and your diaphragm, as it affects both your sacral and lumbar spines, so you know it's a place of personal power and home to the "fire in the belly" that fuels the digestive system and burns up energetic impurities. Not to confuse you, but there is actually a second name for the Manipura chakra—the *Nabhi* chakra, which translates from Sanskrit as "navel wheel."

In yogic philosophy, the Nabhi chakra is considered one of the most sacred places in the body—even among all the revered chakras. It is the place from which many of the 72,000 nadis, or rivers of energy, originate and branch out, supplying energy to your entire body. The Yoga Sutras of Patanjali tell us that a yogi who meditates on the Nabhi chakra "can develop intimate knowledge . . . and can understand everything about the inner workings of the body."[7] Now do you see a new reason to "contemplate your navel"?

Granted, the claims found in the ancient yogic texts often sound far-fetched and out of sync with our present-day lives—some such texts state that if you practice a certain yoga pose, you will be free from all diseases and can safely eat poison! Such claims are not, of course, to be taken literally. But when I think "outside the text," I become quite curious about what the ancient yogis discovered in their practices, and I want to know about my body what they knew about theirs.

Practicing yoga with mindfulness on the Nabhi chakra, the navel wheel, can especially help you gain this type of insight. You may come to understand why you stand a certain way, why you habitually collapse here or protect there, where you carry stress and tension—and most importantly, how you can undo unhealthy postures and habits.

So let's contemplate our navels. Have you ever had what you'd describe as a "knot" in your stomach, when you were nervous or angry perhaps? According to yoga philosophy this feeling is called a *granthi*, which translates as "knot or hardening." Another translation I like is that a granthi is a "complaint." When you experience a granthi, your body is talking to you, complaining that something is stuck! It's your job to help it become unstuck so that your prana, life force, flows freely through the Sushumna energy channel and rises up toward the crown of your head.

One of the most common granthis, the *Brahma granthi*, lies directly inside the navel region. This is no coincidence—in Hindu theology, Brahma is the manifestation of universal energy and the creator of the cosmos. Similarly, your navel is the source of creation in your physical body because it was your lifeline—through the umbilical cord—when you were in your mother's womb.

Your abdominal area is home to a number of Ayurvedic marma points, the energetic points that sit along your nadis. A diagram of these points would look somewhat like a constellation. There's one at the center of your navel, appropriately called the Nabhi point, and four more points that radiate diagonally outward from there. According to Ayurvedic science, stimulation of the Nabhi points kindles your inner fire (*agni* in Sanskrit), regulates all the functions of the abdominal organs, relieves abdominal pain, and stimulates digestion and elimination.[8] This might sound familiar, and it should, because the profound work of the abdominal marma points is similar to the influence of the vagus nerve we discussed earlier in this chapter.

To complete our Eastern view of the abdominal core, let's revisit the concept of *agni*. According to the Ayurvedic tradition, agni is the fire of digestion and metabolism that exists in every cell, every nadi, and every internal organ in your body. It regulates body temperature, aids in digestion and the absorption of food, and transforms food into energy.[9] Yoga practice aims to awaken and balance the intensity of agni so your metabolism and digestion become even and stable.

Agni mainly resides at the lower end of the Sushumna energy channel. But it also combines with the energy of the abdominal area, where it's called *Jathara agni* (stomach fire), and rises up through the whole Sushumna. As it moves up toward the crown of the head, your fiery agni burns up energetic impurities as you inhale and releases them as you exhale, cleansing and purifying your energetic body and bringing both your body and mind to a place of clarity.

Uniting East and West: The Holistic View

Now we'll turn to a concept from the Yoga Sutras of Patanjali to help you see your abdominal core as a powerful meeting place of your physical and energetic bodies. Yoga Sutra 2.1 discusses the concept of *tapas*—"austerity" or "purification" in Sanskrit—as one of the main components of what the text refers to as "the yoga of action."[10] The Sanskrit word *tapas* also translates as "heat, burning, that which burns all impurities, self-discipline."[11]

Since we've already discussed the heat of agni, you can probably quickly see that there's no better place in the body to pursue tapas than the abdominal core. In this chapter, you will notice more meditative practices than in previous chapters. That's because in addition to physical poses that will tone and strengthen your abdominal core, we're after the heat, the profound focus and discipline, that will keep you strong in your innermost core as well as your physical midsection. In short, we're after tapas.

In the context of yoga practice, tapas is the motivation that gets you onto your mat and keeps you there despite the unrelenting tug of iPads and text messages. It's the inspiration that led you to take your first steps toward wellness. It's the reason you opened this book. Tapas generates inner heat and the self-discipline to allow yourself—both your body and your mind—to become refined. Your mind quiets and you can access your inner self, the part of yourself that is larger than who you think you are. You can access, if I may, your very core. Practice your yoga with this kind of focused attention on your inner self, and your experience will become deep and rich, a living meditation on the path to oneness and wellness.

I said earlier in this chapter that we aren't chasing a six-pack abdominal area, chiseled by countless crunches and sit-ups. I meant it! As you work your way through the meditations and exercises in this chapter, remember that what we're really looking for is healthy, disciplined progress toward abdominal tone. *Healthy* really is the operative word, because it is possible, even easy, to overdo abdominal work, leaving you at risk of overtightening your psoas muscles, pulling your lumbar spine into lordosis, or worse. If you're in a rush to achieve some standard of abdominal "perfection," you really aren't in a good place to give your body the gift of tone, balance, and wellness. So proceed mindfully, and carry this mantra with you throughout your practice: Do your best, then rest!

And stay in touch with your inner fire. Your practice starts with a Fire Meditation that will connect you to your agni. When you practice the poses in the rest of the chapter, remember to focus on the flow of your breath and energy in your abdominal area in order to feel the heat you created, and let it help you concentrate and purify your source of personal power. I hope that along your journey you'll find what can be a profound mixture of the physical energy that tones your abdominal core and the vital energy that tones and purifies your internal organs and energetic channels.

Yoga Poses for a Healthy Abdominal Core

Ask and Listen: Preparation for Practice

Fire Meditation

Sit comfortably on your mat or on a blanket with your legs crossed. Your legs and hips should be relaxed. If there is tension in your inner thighs or abdomen, support your knees with blocks. Relax your shoulders and neck. Feel free to sit against a wall for extra support.

Place your hands on your abdomen. Inhaling through your nose, mindfully observe as your breath moves down through your throat and chest, into your abdomen, and down into your hips. Feel your whole abdomen gently expand and spread outward. Exhale completely from your hips through your abdomen, up through your chest and throat, then out through your nose. Feel your abdomen gently softening back toward your spine. Feel each of the next three breaths deepening and lengthening, until you feel your whole abdominal cavity filling with prana as you inhale and completely emptying as you exhale.

Visualize your inner fire, your agni, as a flame born in your abdominal area—a beautiful elliptical light that illuminates your inner self. As you inhale, visualize the flame pointing down toward your hips, and as you exhale, visualize the flame turning upward toward your chest and throat and out your nose, following the flow of your breath. With each inhalation, visualize yourself "fueling your fire" and watch its flame consume the impurities in your body. With each exhalation, visualize releasing the ash of what has been burned out of your body as the flow of your exhalation turns the flame upward and out into the clean, fresh air of the room.

Repeat this Fire Meditation for ten to twelve breaths. With each new breath visualize your body becoming a clean, clear vessel of life force.

"Knit–Your-Abdomen" Meditation

Now you'll explore how to find and engage your abdominal muscles, layer by layer. Lie down with your knees bent and your feet flat on the floor. Your lower back should be comfortable; if it isn't, support it as shown in the Deep Hip Meditation on page 42. Place your hands on your abdomen.

Layer 1: Rectus Abdominis

Keeping your hips on the floor, lift the tip of your tailbone slightly upward, just enough to angle your pubic bone toward your navel, shortening the distance between them. Feel your lower abdomen and navel moving down toward the floor. Then shorten the distance between your navel and your lower ribs. You should start to feel the rectus abdominis—the long muscles that run from your pubic bone to your breastbone—becoming active and engaged.

Layers 2 and 3: Obliques

Perhaps you remember that earlier in this chapter I used the image of your abdominal wall muscles acting like woven layers of mesh that support your abdominal organs and lower back. Now imagine that you are "knitting" back and forth across your abdomen, drawing the fronts of your hip bones toward each other so that the front of your pelvis narrows, and drawing your lower ribs toward one another to narrow the distance between the right and left lower ribs. The layers of mesh should knit together and feel snug without a feeling of muscular gripping (you should be able to breathe with ease). With this action, you will access the next two layers of muscles, the external and internal obliques. These are the muscles that run diagonally across your abdomen and connect your ribs and your hip bones. When they become engaged, you can feel your abdominal wall moving toward its center—your navel.

Slowly straighten your legs one at a time while you maintain the knitting action of your abdominals. (If you placed a folded blanket under your lower back, you'll need to take it away.) When you lie down flat, feel that with your abdominals engaged, your lower back's arch is elongated rather than overdone, and that it is supported by the actions of the abdominals.

Before you explore the deepest layer of abdominal muscles in the next step, take a moment to check in with your lower back. If it is comfortable and happy, you are good to go. If not, return to the bent-knee position and keep your feet on the floor. You'll skip layer 4 until your lower back feels comfortable. In the meantime, you can enjoy the feeling of your abdominal core becoming alive and active by finding layers 1, 2, and 3.

Layer 4: Transversus Abdominis

To find the deepest layer of abdominal muscles, remain lying down with your legs stretched straight on the floor. Ground your buttocks, press out through your heels, and engage your thigh muscles as if you were about to lift your legs up off the floor.[12] Remember to keep your tailbone lifting slightly up. Can you feel how your abdominal wall becomes active from one side to the other? This feeling is the transversus abdominis muscle, the deepest layer of musculature that runs from your lumbar and thoracic spines around each side of your trunk to the front, forming the "belt" that supports your abdominal organs.

Hold these actions for ten seconds and feel the power you've accessed in your abdominal core. Relax for a few breaths. Repeat this exercise a few times so you get used to accessing your core strength. Have you ever journeyed so deeply into your abdominal muscles? As you practice the poses ahead, you'll feel how doing so gives you new access to your core strength in a variety of yoga poses, not to mention in your daily life.

Practice for a Healthy Abdominal Core

The poses in this section are progressive, meaning each one requires slightly more abdominal tone than the last. So you should think of this chapter as a work-in-progress, building strength and ability as you go. Proceed slowly, only moving into the stronger poses when you feel that your abdominals have strengthened enough to support the work of that pose. Come out of any pose if you experience discomfort in your lower back and rest in Child's Pose or Happy Baby Pose (see pages 61 and 93). If you need to let go of a pose that's too challenging for now, do just that—let it go. You'll be able to practice it in the future when your abdominals get stronger.

As a bridge between the abdominal connections you made in our "Ask and Listen" meditations and the physical poses we'll now move through, let's practice some pranayama, or yogic breathwork, in order to continue to kindle the fire of your abdominal core.

Shining-Skull Breath

Kapalabhati Pranayama

Shining-Skull Breath is called *Kapalabhati* in Sanskrit (*kapala* means "skull" and *bhati* means "luster"). This breath earns its name because it cleanses the energetic channels of the body from your hips all the way up to the crown of your head. It's considered both a pranayama practice and a *kriya,* or cleansing practice. Both this breath and Bellows Breath, which you'll practice next, activate and invigorate the abdominal muscles and organs and stimulate digestion.[13]

Sit comfortably on the floor or on a folded blanket. If your back aches, sit against a wall or in a chair. Place both hands on your abdomen. Take a short, quiet inhalation through your nose and exhale forcefully and audibly through your nose by pressing your abdominal wall inward. After a brief, one-second pause, repeat the sequence. Try it a few times until you get the feel of how your abdomen should feel in the pose, then rest your hands on your thighs with your index fingers and thumbs together in Jnana mudra, "the seal of knowledge."

Once you get the hang of it, you can practice anywhere between twelve and twenty rounds of Shining-Skull Breath at a time. After your last round, take a deep, long Ocean Breath inhalation (page 12) through your nose; hold your breath for two to three seconds, and exhale deeply and slowly with Ocean Breath. Practice two more rounds of Shining-Skull Breath. Always finish each set with a full Ocean Breath to rest your lungs and cool your brain. After you've finished, sit quietly and observe your body. Go inside and feel how you've awakened your inner energy and stimulated your body and your mind in a healthy, positive way. You might actually feel tired in your abdominal muscles, as if you had done some of those much-maligned crunches! Enjoy this sensation, and know that you've done something kind and invigorating for your abdominal core.

Bellows Breath

Bhastrika Pranayama

Bellows Breath generates prana and activates the energy of the entire body.[14] It gets its name because the abdominal muscles draw air into the body and then push it back out, like a bellows. The fire imagery continues with this practice—a bellows stokes a fire by pumping evenly to forcefully pull air in and push it out. Thus, unlike in Shining-Skull Breath, the inhalation and exhalation in Bellows Breath are *both* very powerful.

Because of its intensity, a word of caution is appropriate. A two- or three-minute Bellows Breath practice ignites plenty of heat and activity in your body, and that's all you need for a healthy practice. Overdoing strong breath practices such as Bellows and Shining Skull can endanger your lungs, cause dizziness, and fatigue your body.

Sit comfortably, as you did for Shining-Skull breath. Place your hands on your abdomen. Take one deep, long preparatory breath with a deep inhalation and a long exhalation. To start Bellows Breath, inhale sharply and forcefully through your nose. You should feel your abdominal wall press out into your hands. Then forcefully exhale, pulling your abdominal wall inward to push your breath out. You've just completed one round of Bellows Breath. All the action comes from your abdominal area—keep your upper chest and your shoulders relaxed. Practice a few rounds until you are comfortable with the breath.

Practice between twelve and twenty rounds in a row of Bellows Breath. Follow it with a long Ocean Breath inhalation; hold your breath in for two to three seconds, then release a long Ocean Breath exhalation. Sit quietly afterward. If your body is comfortable, practice two more sets of Bellows Breath, each set followed by a full Ocean Breath to rest your lungs. You should feel very warm afterward, with a feeling that you've completely awakened your abdominal core, your energetic body, and your inner fire.

Earlier in this chapter I talked about the Brahma granthi, the energetic knot that forms at the navel area and inhibits the flow of energy up the Sushumna, the central energy channel of the body. In yogic philosophy, Bellows Breath pierces the Brahma granthi and opens the energy of the Nabhi chakra, the navel wheel. Not only that, Bellows opens two other energetic knots, the Vishnu granthi, located at the Anahata chakra, or heart center, and the Rudra granthi, located at the Ajna chakra, or third eye.[15] By cracking open these granthis, Bellows Breath allows energy to flow freely and completely up through the Sushumna, from the base of the hips to the crown of the head.

If I may get philosophical for a moment, it's significant that these knots are named after the three major manifestations of universal energy in yogic philosophy—Brahma, the creator; Vishnu, the preserver; and Rudra (another name for Shiva), the destroyer. Perhaps the ancient yogis accessed incredible stores of energy with Bellows Breath. This might sound to you like another one of those outlandish claims that the yogis tended to make, but when you practice Bellows Breath . . . well, perhaps you can find a little bit of that power within yourself!

Table-Balance Tuck Pose

Stretch and Strengthen | Vyaghrasana Variation 2

Start in Cat Pose (page 45). Lift your navel strongly up toward the ceiling and draw your tailbone and your head downward and toward each other. Hold this position for one or two breaths and feel your abdomen knitting together as we practiced earlier. This is a moving pose, so you will need to be mindful of your abdominal knit in order to get its full benefits.

Step 1: Three-Legged Table Tuck

While in Cat Pose, exhale and draw your right knee into your chest (fig. 5.1). As you inhale, slowly and mindfully stretch your right leg back and up until it is parallel to the floor; lift your head and shoulders to look forward.

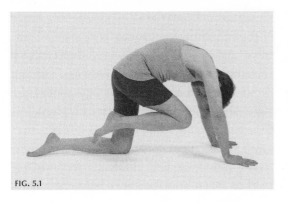

FIG. 5.1

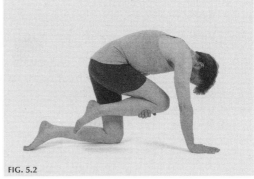

FIG. 5.2

As you exhale, come back into Cat Pose with your right knee tucked in to your chest. Practice this movement three times to each side, using deep breaths to guide your movements. Keep your abdominal wall engaged while you inhale and stretch your leg up and back.

Step 2: Table-Balance Tuck

The final pose requires more core stability than Three-Legged Table Tuck because you will balance on one hand and one leg. If you were comfortable in that pose, you're ready for it.

Start again in Cat Pose. As you exhale, draw your right knee into your chest and reach your left arm under your trunk to touch your right shin with your left hand (fig. 5.2). As you inhale, stretch your right leg up and back and reach your left arm forward and up, coming into Table-Balance Pose. Remember to keep your abdomen knitted together! Repeat this step two more times balancing on your left shin and right hand. Rest in Child's Pose for a few breaths before you practice it three times with the opposite arm and leg, and rest again in Child's Pose when you're done.

High Plank Pose

Strengthen | Phalakasana

In High Plank Pose, you'll knit your abdomen together while you support your body on just your hands and feet. You'll need to work strongly through your arms and legs to support the weight of your body.

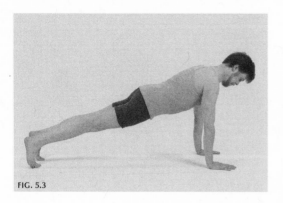

FIG. 5.3

Start in Downward-Facing Dog Pose (page 145), stretching up through your arms, shoulders, and hips and stretching your legs down toward the floor. On an exhalation, keeping your legs straight, drop your hips about halfway down to the floor and shift your trunk forward until your shoulders are directly over your wrists (fig. 5.3). Draw your navel up toward your spine and knit your abdomen together. Keep your abdomen and chest long, draw your shoulder blades away from your neck, and lengthen your breastbone forward. Feel that your body is an even, upward-sloping plank from your ankles through your hips and shoulders, all the way to your head.

Hold for ten to fifteen seconds, place your knees on the floor, and rest in Child's Pose. Return to Down Dog and repeat High Plank Pose two more times, focusing on using the firmness in your abdomen and the strength of your arms and legs to support your body. High Plank builds arm and leg tone while it strengthens your core.

Note: If you have a shoulder injury or any other condition that prevents you from supporting yourself comfortably in the pose, there are two quick modifications that you can try. You can either place your knees on the floor, or practice the pose with your forearms on the floor rather than bearing weight on your wrists. Any way you practice High Plank Pose will strengthen your abdomen.

Upward-Legs Pose

Strengthen | Urdhva Prasarita Padasana

Step 1: Supported Upward-Legs Pose

Lie on your back with your feet flat on the floor and a belt within reach. Exhaling, draw your knees into your chest and place the belt around your feet. With your next exhalation, stretch your legs straight up toward the ceiling, or bend your knees slightly if you can't comfortably hold your legs perpendicular to your body. Hold your belt with your arms straight and your shoulders relaxed (fig. 5.4).

Keep your hips on the floor, lift your tailbone upward as if you could lift it all the way up to your feet, and knit your abdomen together. These actions will help your lower back stay supported and comfortable.

Step 2: Full Upward-Legs Pose

Leaving your legs raised, put your belt aside, then reach your arms all the way up over your head to the floor. If you feel any amount of discomfort in your back, place your hands under your hips instead; if that doesn't relieve your

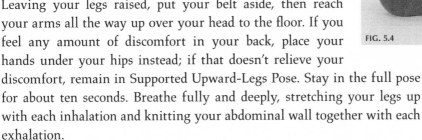
FIG. 5.4

discomfort, remain in Supported Upward-Legs Pose. Stay in the full pose for about ten seconds. Breathe fully and deeply, stretching your legs up with each inhalation and knitting your abdominal wall together with each exhalation.

To come out, bend your knees back into your chest and hug them for a few moments, then move your legs gently from side to side to massage your lower back. Rest your legs flat on the floor and relax for a few breaths.

Place your hands on your abdomen and feel the warmth and energy you have created in your core. Be particularly mindful of your psoas (hip flexor) muscle, which can feel overworked or tight after this pose. For most practitioners, lying with legs flat on the floor and breathing down into the hips is enough to release the tension after practicing this pose. But if your psoas muscles are tight to begin with, proceed through these poses with mindful caution.

Upward-Legs Curl-Up

Strengthen | Urdhva Prasarita Padasana Variation 1

If your lower back is comfortable in Full Upward-Legs Pose, you're ready to progress into Upward-Legs Curl-Up. Otherwise, see below for modifications that will help you practice the pose with greater comfort.

Start in Upward-Legs Pose with your arms over your head. As you

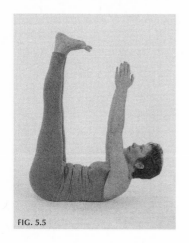

FIG. 5.5

exhale, lift your arms up toward the ceiling (not trying to touch your toes) and curl your shoulders and head up off the floor (fig. 5.5). Hold yourself up for two seconds, and as you inhale, bring your shoulders, head, and arms back down to the floor. Repeat the pose, curling up again with your next exhalation.

Upward-Legs Curl-Up is a brisk pose—move in and out of it fairly quickly, following your natural inhalations and exhalations. Practice three repetitions at first and then come out; make sure your lower back is comfortable. Increase the repetitions as you feel stronger, cycling through the pose up to ten times.

If your back needs more support in this pose, keep one foot grounded on the floor. Practice four or five repetitions to one side, then change legs and repeat to the opposite side. For even more support, keep both feet on the ground. If your neck feels strained when you lift your shoulders and head off the floor, support your head with your hands.

To come out of the pose, hug your knees into your chest for a few moments and then rest with your legs flat on the floor, again taking care to note the condition and comfort of your lower back.

Active Bent-Knee Twist

Stretch and Strengthen | Jathara Parivartanasana Variation 2

After a pose such as Upward-Legs Curl-Up, a simple lying twist feels delicious, because the abdominals get a good stretch and any tension in them is released. You'll "taste" that in a minute, but before you do, you'll practice a version that strengthens and tones your internal and external oblique muscles. Trust me, this will make your "just dessert" even sweeter!

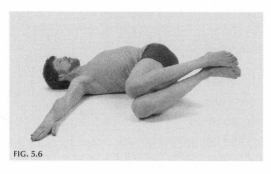

Lie on the floor and draw your knees to your chest. Stretch your arms out to the sides even with your shoulders. Turn your palms down. Feel your upper back and shoulders fully grounded on the floor. Take a deep inhalation and feel your chest broadening, and as you exhale, slowly take your legs down to the right, keeping your knees and feet together as you go. Bring your right thigh and knee down

FIG. 5.6

to the floor, but keep your right shin and foot off the floor (fig. 5.6). Your left shoulder should stay grounded. If your knee can't reach the floor or if your lower back is in discomfort, support your right knee on a block.

Draw your outer left hip away from your waist and draw your lower back muscles in toward your abdomen. You'll feel some muscular effort along the sides of your trunk—these are the external and internal oblique muscles we've discussed. Also, see if you can feel your lower back lengthening and releasing. Turn your head to look at your left hand, and stay in the pose for a few breaths. With an inhalation, bring your legs back up to center and repeat to the opposite side as you exhale. Repeat again to each side.

Relaxing Bent-Knee Twist

Rest | Jathara Parivartanasana Variation 3

If Bent-Knee Twist is comfortable in your lower back, you can practice it now as a resting pose . . . the delicious "dessert" I promised you! Begin as above, but now take your whole right leg down to the floor or onto a block, whichever your body prefers. Stay for a few breaths and enjoy the feeling of length and release in your abdomen and lower back. You can deepen the twist by pressing your right hand down on your left thigh and turning your torso more to the left.

To come out of this resting version, draw your knees up to your armpit before you bring them back to the center. Take a deep inhalation as you lift your legs up, and with an exhalation repeat the pose to the opposite side. If your lower back feels tight, you can choose to practice Reclining Bolster Twist (page 154) instead. Or, release your lower back and soften your abdomen for a few moments in Happy Baby Pose (page 93).

Deep Relaxation: Illuminate Your Core

Rest | Shavasana Variation 4

As we prepare to deeply relax at the end of our practice, I'd like to introduce a yogic idea that will help you rest into all we've done for your abdominal core so far.

One goal of yoga practice is to balance the three qualities of nature that exist in everything in the universe, including your own body. These qualities, or *gunas* in Sanskrit, are:

- *Tamas:* inertia, rest, and darkness
- *Rajas:* movement, activity, and passion
- *Sattva:* equanimity and illumination

I'm sure you've experienced all three of these qualities in yourself at various times. Sometimes it's clear which guna is predominant, such as when you're having a really lazy day (tamas), or when you've got an extraordinary amount of energy (rajas). At other times you've probably felt that your energy level is a mix of rest, action, and the interplay between them.

When the gunas are balanced, the quality of sattva becomes predominant and the practitioner moves into a state of physical and mental equilibrium. In such a balanced state, he isn't affected by the push and pull of tamas and rajas, and according to the Yoga Sutras of Patanjali, he "comes to experience his own soul with crystal clarity."[16]

The gunas have an important relationship to the abdominal area. Tamas resides in the lower abdomen and hips, and rajas lives between the navel and heart. Abdominal practices wake up tamas, that dark, resting inertia. As Kundalini energy uncoils and the energy of the lower body rises up into the chest, tamas unites with rajas, the quality of passionate, active movement. Together, the two gunas travel up through the spine; when they reach the top of your head at the crown (Sahasrara) chakra, they turn into sattva, illumination.

As you relax, I'll take you through a visualization of these qualities—how they awaken, how they move through your hips and abdomen and up through your body to your head, and how they turn into the light that illuminates the path to your true nature.

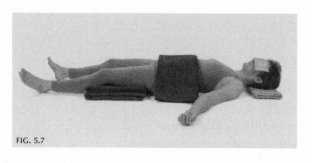

FIG. 5.7

Lie down comfortably on your mat or on a blanket. Place a folded blanket under your thighs with the top edge of the blanket at your upper thighs. You should feel your lower back lengthening. If your sacrum is in discomfort, support it with a folded towel. Place another folded blanket across your abdomen as a reminder for it to relax. Support your

YOGA FOR A HEALTHY LOWER BACK

head so your neck is comfortable, and place an eye pillow over your eyes as a reminder for your eyes to quiet down and look within (fig. 5.7).

Inhale down into your belly, feeling it expand gently upward while you visualize the skin, layers of myofascia, and layers of muscles lengthening and opening. Visualize all those layers relaxing down into the earth as you exhale. Take a few breaths and let the energy of your abdomen become quiet and settled.

Visualize the inner fire and heat you created as you practiced the exercises in this chapter as a luminous elliptical light in your abdomen. Now that your inner fire is lit (and is nice and hot), let it break through the dullness and darkness (the tamas guna) that tends to settle into your hips. Visualize that inner fire awakening the serpentine Kundalini energy that lies in wait at the base of your spine. Visualize Kundalini energy as a beautiful, luminous light winding up through the central channel of the spine from your sacral chakra to your lower back, carrying rajas, the quality of movement that we used in our practice, into your upper body and head. When the light reaches your head, let it become pure illumination, sattva, making your mind clear and pure. Let the light linger in your head for a few moments and visualize its radiance.

Now visualize the light slowly moving back down your body, all the way to the base of your spine. Feel yourself fully grounded to the earth. Feel the energy of your body perfectly balanced between rest and action and between darkness and light. Feel your mind balanced, and visualize your light illuminating your path of awareness.

Grow and Progress

Reawaken Your Fire: Abdominal Lock

Uddiyana Bandha

You practiced Root Lock, or Mula Bandha, in chapter 2 (page 39), lifting your perineal floor and lower abdomen in and up toward your spine. Now you'll find the strong energetic lock called Uddiyana Bandha, or Abdominal Lock. In Sanskrit, *uddiyana* means "flying up" or "soaring"—and that's just the way it feels, as if your abdomen and everything in it were soaring up into your chest. Uddiyana Bandha tones the abdomen, increases inner fire, and

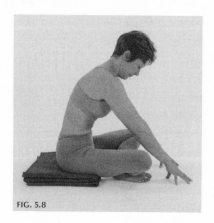

helps to flush toxins out of your inner organs.[17] Energetically speaking, Abdominal Lock cleans out the residue of what is burned up by your inner fire.

Uddiyana Bandha can be practiced either standing up or sitting down. I'll teach it to you in a seated position so you can feel your hips grounded to the earth and the strong upward lift in your abdomen. You'll see that it makes sense to practice Abdominal Lock only on an empty stomach. It's contraindicated for abdominal pain or inflammation, fever, during the menstrual cycle, and during late pregnancy.

Sit up tall on your mat in a cross-legged position. You'll need to be able to bend forward easily from your hip joints and keep the front of your trunk long, so if your knees are higher than your groins or if your lower back is collapsing, sit on a folded blanket or bolster.

Lift your arms up and take a deep, full inhalation. As you quickly and forcefully exhale, reach your arms down to the floor in front of your trunk and place your fingertips on the floor (or on blocks if your hips are on a bolster). Look down, but do not allow your head and chest to collapse into a full forward bend. Hold your breath without inhaling while you strongly draw your whole abdominal area back toward your spine and up toward your chest (fig. 5.8). Lift your trunk, tuck your chin slightly (but keep your upper chest open), and roll your shoulders back. Hold Abdominal Lock only as long as your endurance allows—you shouldn't feel any pressure or tension in your eyes, tongue, or temples.

Release Abdominal Lock, take a deep, full inhalation, then return to sitting upright. Take a few normal breaths and observe the powerful effect Uddiyana Bandha has had on your energetic body. Repeat Abdominal Lock two more times. After you're finished, lie down on your back with your hands on your abdomen and visualize the energy of your lower body and upper body combined, the two energies becoming consistent, uniform, and pure.

Reclining Leg Circles

Strengthen | Urdhva Prasarita Padasana Variation 2

Start in Upward-Legs Pose (page 186) with your head cradled in your hands, or place your hands under your hips to support your lower back. Keep your

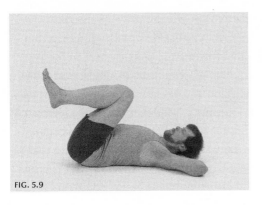

FIG. 5.9

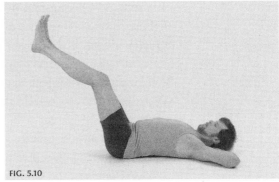

FIG. 5.10

abdominal wall knitted together and firm. Exhaling, bend your knees slightly toward your chest (fig. 5.9). With an inhalation reach your legs away from your chest (fig. 5.10) and lift them up toward the ceiling, bringing them back to the vertical position (fig. 5.11).

You've now completed one Reclining Leg Circle. Practice a few times by tracing small circles in the air with your feet, imagining you are pedaling a bicycle that has only one pedal. If your lower back feels comfortable, make the circles a little bigger. Practice five or six circles and bring your knees into your chest to rest for a few moments.

Now you'll change the direction of your circles. From your starting position in Upward-Legs Pose, take your feet away from your body as you exhale. Inhaling, bend your knees and bring them toward your chest, and finish your circle by reaching your legs back up to the ceiling as you exhale. Repeat five or six circles in this direction, tracing larger circles if your lower back is comfortable. When you are done, rest with your knees into your chest, gently moving them from to side to side to massage your sacrum.

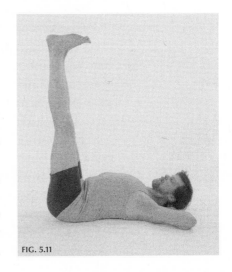

You can feel the strengthening power of Reclining Leg Circles by resting your legs down on the floor and placing your hands on your pelvis when you're finished. Feel the warmth in your hips and sense the energy you have created there.

As you rest after this pose, let me briefly introduce a concept from Taoism, the Chinese religion mostly known through the writings of the ancient teachers

FIG. 5.11

Your Abdominal Core

Lao-tzu and Chuang-tzu. In Taoist philosophy, all movements that stimulate the lower abdominal area invigorate the physical and energetic center of gravity in your body called the *xia dantian*.[18]

This energetic focal point is a place of deep inner strength and peace, a combination of physical, energetic, and emotional grounding and fluidity. Each of our body's three *dantians*, meaning "seas of energy," is a focal point of chi (vital energy) in the body. It's not a coincidence that the lower dantian corresponds almost exactly with the yogic notion of Svadhisthana chakra, the place where prana (life force) gathers. As one Taoist states, "The more life force one has, the stronger and healthier one is bound to become."[19] All the more reason to invest the time and energy in toning, invigorating, and strengthening your abdominal core!

Leg-Lifts Cycle

Strengthen | Urdhva Prasarita Padasana Vinyasa

Leg-Lifts Cycle is a rigorous *vinyasa*, a cycle of sequential movements, requiring a good amount of abdominal stability in order to maintain comfort in your lower back. You'll practice this sequence step by step, starting with your knees bent and progressing to lifting one straight leg at a time; finally, if your lower back is agreeable, you'll practice it with both legs straight and lifting together.

Steps 1 through 3 are not yoga poses per se; rather, they are important preparatory steps to ready your body for step 4, the yoga pose called Two-Legs Lift (with Straight Legs). Practice each step the same way you practice any yoga pose—with mindful attention and continuous, deep breathing—and you'll build tone in your abdominal core while your mind stays cool and calm. Be sure to rest between each step and listen to the feedback of your lower back. Practice each of the next steps only when you feel ready.

I am instructing you to exhale when you lift your legs up and when you take them down—that's because I believe practicing both movements that way is the key to a leg lift that fully engages the abdominal muscles. It's much easier to draw your navel down toward your spine and knit your abdominal wall together on an exhalation, and breathing out also helps keep your lower back long, reducing your chance of straining your lower back or overusing your psoas (hip flexor) muscles. After you've practiced each step, take a few moments to rest with your legs flat on the floor to release any tension in your psoas muscles, then hug your knees to your chest for a few breaths before moving on to the next step.

Step 1: One-Leg Lift (with Other Leg Bent)

Lie on your back with your legs bent and your feet flat on the floor. Place your arms overhead on the floor or take your hands under your hips for more lower back support. As you exhale, draw your right knee into your chest and lift your leg straight up so it is perpendicular to your body (fig. 5.12). With your next exhalation, lower your right leg straight down to the floor. Rest for a few breaths and reverse the steps, lifting your leg back to the ceiling and bending your knee into your chest as you exhale. Repeat three times with each leg.

Step 2: One-Leg Lift (with Other Leg Straight)

Repeat step 1, this time with your nonlifting leg flat on the floor. Keep your "down" leg active by pressing out through your heel and drawing your toes toward your knee. And although I might sound like a broken record, I'll say it again: before you begin the pose, knit your abdominal wall together any amount possible. Repeat three times with each leg.

Step 3: Two-Legs Lift (with Knees Bent)

Lie on your back with your legs bent and feet flat on the floor. If you feel confident in the strength of your lower back, straighten your arms onto the

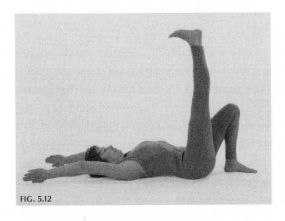

FIG. 5.12

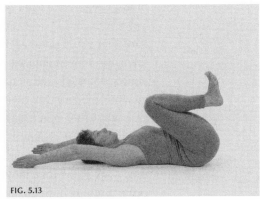

FIG. 5.13

floor behind your head. Otherwise, place your hands, palms down, underneath your hips. As you exhale, bring your knees one at a time into your chest (fig. 5.13). Hold them there as you inhale, and with your next exhalation straighten them both up to the ceiling. Keep your knees bent if any discomfort comes while you're straightening your legs. Inhaling, bring your knees back into your chest, and with your next exhalation, stretch your legs straight out along the floor with your toes pointed to the ceiling. With your next exhalation, bend your knees and place your feet flat on the floor, coming back to your starting position. Repeat Bent-Leg Lift two more times.

Step 4: Two-Legs Lift (with Straight Legs)

This is the most challenging step in the cycle, and caution is advised. Your lower back should feel absolutely comfortable in the previous steps before you practice this step. If you experience twinges or discomfort anywhere in your lower back, release the pose immediately. Practice steps 1 through 3 until your abdominals strengthen.

Lie on your back with your legs flat on the floor. Place your arms overhead on the floor or take your hands under your hips to support your lower back. You may wish to place a folded blanket under your hips. Take a deep inhalation and as you exhale, lift your legs up to ninety degrees from the floor. Hold your legs up as you inhale, and as you exhale, take your legs straight down to the floor. Repeat three times.

One-Legged Downward-Facing Dog Pose

Strengthen | Eka Pada Adho Mukha Svanasana

Now that you've learned Three-Legged Table Tuck (page 184), you'll practice the same movements while in Downward-Facing Dog to strengthen both your abdominals and your lumbar spine muscles. Before you do, though, review and practice Downward-Facing Dog Pose (page 145) until you feel strong and stable; then you're ready to proceed into One-Legged Dog.

Begin in Downward-Facing Dog Pose. Tuck your right knee into your chest and with an exhalation, lift it back and up. Bend your right knee, letting your right foot move toward your left buttock (fig. 5.14). Lift your right thigh as high as possible, until you feel a good stretch all along the

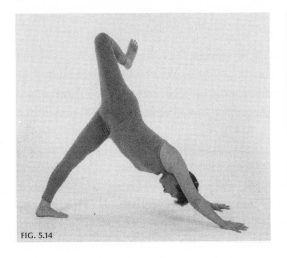

FIG. 5.14

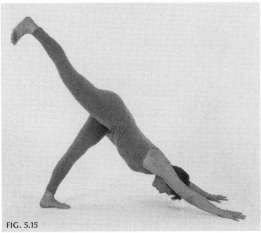

FIG. 5.15

right side of your trunk. Now stretch your right leg straight, forming a single, angled line from your hands to your right foot (fig. 5.15). Engaging your abdominal core is the key to coming into a comfortable One-Legged Dog Pose—it will help you lift your weight out of your wrists and shoulders, and you'll find a great feeling of length and expansion through your spine. Hold the pose for five to ten seconds, and then rest in Child's Pose (page 61) when you're done.

Boat Pose Cycle

Strengthen | Paripurna Navasana Vinyasa

In Boat Pose, your body forms a V-shape with your hips on the floor and your legs and trunk angled upward. This is considered a challenging abdominal pose because all your abdominal core and back muscles are involved in supporting your trunk, and tone and mobility are required in your hamstrings and hip flexors.

Before you attempt Boat Pose, you'll practice a five-step vinyasa of supported movements. Just like in Leg-Lifts Cycle, these are important preparatory steps to ready your body for Full Boat Pose. Be sure to rest between each step and listen to the feedback of your lower back. Practice all the steps only when you feel ready.

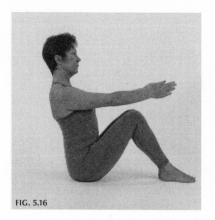

FIG. 5.16

Step 1: Grounded Bent-Knee Pose

Sit on your mat with your legs stretched out in front and your hands on the floor at your sides and behind your hips. Lift your trunk upward and broaden your upper chest. Draw your navel in and up and knit your abdominal wall together, taking care not to overarch your lumbar spine. Draw your shoulder blades away from your neck.

From this strong seated position, bend your knees and place your feet flat on the floor. Be sure to keep your lower back lifting rather than letting it collapse. If that's not possible, sit on a folded blanket to help lift your hips. With an exhalation stretch your arms straight forward, palms facing each other (fig. 5.16). Hold your position for ten to fifteen seconds; breathe smoothly and deeply. Release your arms back down to your sides, straighten your legs, and return to Staff Pose.

Step 2: One-Legged Grounded Bent-Knee Pose

Start in Grounded Bent-Knee Pose (step 1), but this time keep your hands on the floor. As you exhale, stretch your right leg up toward the ceiling, at about a forty-five-degree angle from your hips (fig. 5.17). Hold for one breath, then bring your right foot back down to the floor and stretch your left leg up. Be sure not to let too much weight or pressure come into your hands as you practice this variation. Repeat three times to each side.

Step 3: Bent-Knee Balance

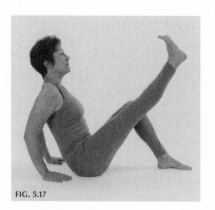

FIG. 5.17

Start the same way you did in step 2. As you exhale, lean back ever so slightly and lift both feet off the floor, with your knees still bent (fig. 5.18). Lift your trunk with each inhalation, and as you exhale, relax your groins down toward the floor. Hold your position for ten to fifteen seconds and remind your body to repeat the actions you've done so far in your chest, shoulder blades, lower back, abdomen, and groins.

When you lift both feet off the floor, you need a little extra grounding through the base of your hips to stabilize your body, so relax your groins, feeling them melt down to the ground, and drop your outer hips to the floor. If you still feel unstable, practice with a folded blanket placed about two inches away from the back of your pelvis so that when you lean back, your sacral joints are supported by the blanket. This blanket support may also be helpful in the remaining steps.

Check in with your lower back. If you're ready for a break, stretch your legs straight onto the floor, or rest in Child's Pose for a few moments before moving on to step 4.

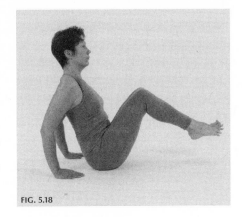
FIG. 5.18

Step 4: One-Legged Supported Boat Pose

Start in Bent-Knee Balance (step 3). Hold your position as you inhale, and as you exhale, lift your right leg up toward the ceiling (fig. 5.19). Hold for one breath, bring your right leg back into Bent-Knee Balance on your next exhalation, then lift your left leg up again, repeating three times to each side.

Step 5: Two-Legged Supported Boat Pose

Start in Bent-Knee Balance (step 3) again. Hold your position as you inhale, and as you exhale slowly stretch both legs up toward the ceiling, either one at a time or, if your lower back is agreeable, stretch them up together (fig. 5.20). Straighten your legs if you can, but keep them bent if it feels too tenuous in your lower back. It may seem like lifting both legs up more than doubles the work . . . and it does. You no longer have the downward position

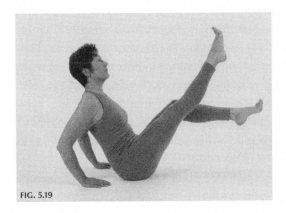
FIG. 5.19

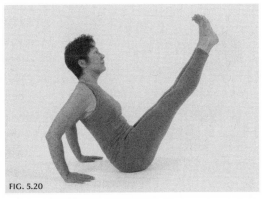
FIG. 5.20

of one bent leg to balance out the work the abdominal and spinal muscles need to do to keep your trunk lifted. Hold the pose for five to ten seconds, breathing deeply and smoothly. To come out of the pose, bend your knees and place your feet back down on the floor, then slowly lie down on your back and relax before practicing Full Boat Pose.

Step 6: Full Boat Pose

Start in Two-Legged Supported Boat Pose (step 5). With an exhalation, take one hand off the ground and stretch your arm straight forward, parallel to the ground. On your next exhalation, stretch your other arm forward and turn your palms toward each other (fig. 5.21). Make sure your lower back is still lifting up as much as possible without tipping into an overarch.

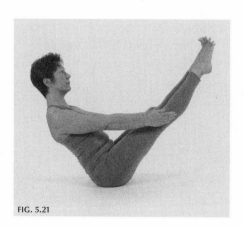

FIG. 5.21

You're finally in the deepest stage of Boat Pose. Breathe deeply. Relax your eyes, throat, and tongue. Lift your trunk with every inhalation, and relax your groins with every exhalation. When your hamstrings are long and your hip flexors are toned, your feet will be higher than your head and your eyes will be gazing straight across at your shins.

Hold Boat Pose as long as your body enjoys its intensity and your lower back feels comfortable, anywhere from five to fifteen seconds. When you are ready to come out, bend your knees and place your feet back on the floor.

Lie down on your back and rest your hands on your lower abdomen. Visualize your abdominals, spinal muscles, and psoas muscles relaxing and softening into the support of the earth. Although pride can sometimes be a deleterious emotion, now is a moment to embrace and celebrate what your body is able to do!

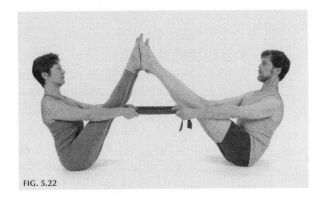

FIG. 5.22

Full Boat Pose, Partner Variation

Before we move on to our last abdominal core pose, try a playful variation of Boat Pose with a partner in order to practice it with more support for your lower back. Sit facing each other in step 1: Grounded Bent-Knee Pose. With your hands on the floor, place the soles of your feet against the soles of your partner's feet, and hold each other's wrists, or hold belts as shown in figure 5.22. Maintain this position for a few breaths while you find your balance, then with an exhalation slowly lift your legs up (all four of them!) toward the ceiling, one side at a time. Remain in the pose for ten to fifteen seconds. Slowly bend your knees, bring your feet back down to the ground, and release your hands.

Half Boat Pose

Strengthen | Ardha Navasana

This may sound backward, but it's true: when you're comfortable in Full Boat Pose, it's beneficial and abdominally strengthening to move from it into Half Boat Pose. In Half Boat, your body forms a slight concave curve rather than the sharp V-form of Full Boat.

Start in Full Boat Pose. When you feel steady, take your hands behind your head and place your fingers lightly on the back of your skull. Your elbows should open out to the sides. Draw your navel down toward your

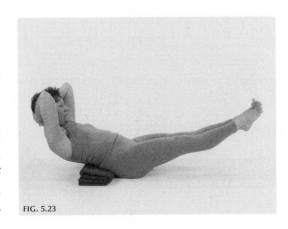

FIG. 5.23

spine and knit your abdominal wall together any amount possible. With your next exhalation, lower your legs almost—but not all the way—to the floor. Now lower your trunk just a bit toward the floor. Keep your lower back off the floor—you should be balanced on your buttocks. Your eyes should gaze straight at your feet (fig. 5.23). If this is a challenging pose for you, place a folded blanket behind your hips before you begin and use it to support your sacral band, as shown in the photo.

Hold Half Boat Pose as long as your body enjoys its fierceness, then lie down on the floor and relax. Place your hands on your abdomen and breathe up into them, feeling your abdominal muscles release any tension that might have crept in during your practice. One more time, congratulate yourself on cultivating strength and tone in your body that will carry you through your life as well as your yoga practice.

Relaxing Bent-Knee Twist, Child's Pose, and Deep Relaxation

Rest | Jathara Parivartanasana Variation 3, Balasana, and Shavasana, Variation 4

Be sure to rest your body after you've completed your abdominal practice. A gentle twist can feel exceptionally good after abdominal poses. Practice Relaxing Bent-Knee Twist (page 189), and Child's Pose (page 61). Then rest in Deep Relaxation for five minutes or longer, resting into the image of the inner fire of your abdominal core, illuminating, warming, and enlivening your whole self.

6

Your Middle Back, Upper Back, and Neck

What does your neck have to do with a healthy lower back? Asking that question is like asking what the roof of a building has to do with its foundation. If the building's foundation is uneven, the roof will be askew and cause leaks, rot, and all sorts of other problems. If the roof is not pitched correctly, those problems will (literally!) trickle down to the foundation, undermining it and potentially putting the whole structure at risk.

The architecture of your body is no different, in this way, from the architecture of a building. We have discussed throughout our journey so far that a healthy spine is a smooth, flowing S-curve. It must, therefore, be clear that your middle back, upper back, and neck—being parts of your spinal column—have a direct relationship to the comfort of your lower back, sacrum, and hips. The curve goes from top to bottom, and every inch of it impacts the whole.

Our work in this chapter starts with taking a long, hard look at your posture. Whatever you do in your personal and professional life affects how you carry yourself. Eating, sitting, driving, reading, carrying children, typing, texting, and sleeping are just a few of the activities that involve your middle back, upper back, and neck. You can probably name a time when you were doing something "normal," like making a bed or tying a shoelace, when all of a sudden a muscle in your upper back or neck went into a twinge, knot, or spasm. If you've had lower back pain for even just a few weeks, you know how your upper back and neck tend to respond—they can overwork to compensate for the lower back and tighten up because of it—and how that affects your movements.

The majority of middle and upper back issues are either cases of myofascial pain from improper postural habits, injuries from overuse or repetitive motion, or spinal joint dysfunction, where a vertebra is abnormally positioned or out of alignment with the rest of the spine.[1] The pain can feel like aching discomfort in the upper back and neck, tenderness around the neck or shoulder blades, or sharp pain that radiates through the neck, upper back, or upper chest and arms. In such cases, you often lose range of motion, especially in the neck and shoulders.[2] Other conditions that produce middle and upper back and neck pain include scoliosis, spinal stenosis, degenerative disk disease and injuries resulting from whiplash.[3]

In this chapter, you'll explore how you can create both fluidity and tone in your middle back, upper back, and neck as a means of support for your journey into lower back health, as well as for their own sake. Because all the parts of your spine are inextricably connected to one another, I'll be referring back to poses you've practiced in other chapters that have additional benefits in your upper back and neck. You'll also learn new poses that will guide your upper back and neck a little farther toward releasing tension and "reshaping" themselves back toward their natural healthy curvatures.

Through Western Eyes: The Physical View

Anatomically speaking, this chapter will complete our journey up the spine, through your thoracic and cervical spines (illustration 17).

The middle and upper back, or thoracic spine, contains twelve vertebrae. It begins at the top of your lumbar spine and grows thinner and narrower as it climbs upward to its meeting point with your cervical spine (neck), just below the tops of your shoulders.

The character of your middle and upper back is quite different from that of your lower back. You may recall that I described your lumbar spine as a flexible stack of bones, with the back of the hip bones to restrict their movement at lumbar vertebra L5. I also mentioned the connection between your lumbar spine and your cervical spine: They both have concave curves—if they're healthy, that is—and more range of motion than the thoracic spine. Because of that, both your lumbar and cervical spines are more vulnerable than your thoracic spine to injuries and painful conditions including herniated disks and degenerative disk disease.

In contrast to the relative freedom of the lumbar and cervical spines, your thoracic spine is well connected to surrounding bones, specifically your ribs and breastbone. Your thoracic spine, ribs, breastbone, and the cartilage that connects the latter two form your rib cage, which surrounds and protects the thoracic cavity and the organs within it, including your heart and lungs. Because of its connections to the ribs and breastbone, your thoracic spine is designed for upright twisting and some forward bending (but not a lot); it has much less range of motion in backbends and side-bending than your lumbar spine does.

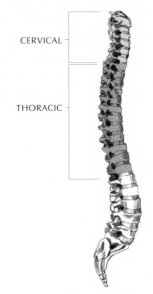

CERVICAL

THORACIC

Illustration 17. Your Thoracic and Cervical Spines

The cervical spine forms the support for your skull. The top cervical vertebra, C1, is the atlas, the base of your skull (remember, spinal vertebrae are numbered from top to bottom). Below C1 is C2, the pivot point upon which C1 rotates. C1 and C2 form the joint that connects your skull with your spine.[4] There are seven cervical vertebrae in all—you can often see or feel C7 as a bony protuberance just below the tops of the shoulders.

The Interconnectedness of Your Spine

As I said before, we'll start by thinking about poor posture, and the havoc it can wreak on your entire back body. We'll look at a few dysfunctional ways many of us hold ourselves, and the respective chains of discomfort those poor postural habits can cause.

Trouble often starts with tight hip flexor (psoas) muscles, which pull the sacral and hip bones forward, tightening up your lower back. As I've noted earlier, this leads to an exaggerated lordosis, which pulls your lower back muscles forward toward your front body. Tight psoas muscles can also pull one or both legs up, which results in a functional leg-length difference, causing further shear in the sacral joints. Because your body is always trying to find its balance, your upper back responds to a lordosis by an exaggerated rounding and hunching of the thoracic spine called a kyphosis. Excessive kyphosis can also be caused by poor postural habits or repetitive strain on the thoracic muscles, such as the shoulders shifting forward in relation to the hips in a seated position—hm, computers, anyone?

While poor posture does not directly cause pain, it does create vulnerability to injury in the middle back, upper back, and neck. Kyphosis causes the shoulder blades to slide away from the spine, chronically overstretching and weakening the muscles around the shoulder blades.[5] It has a profound effect on the front of your chest as well, shortening and tightening the myofascia of the upper chest, which then pulls on your upper back and neck muscles again, overstretching and weakening the myofascia even further. The spaces around your heart, lungs, and diaphragm then become constricted and tight. Because your body is still trying to bring itself into balance, your head shifts forward, creating tension and tightness in your neck muscles. Keep this in mind throughout this chapter, especially as you practice both active and supported backbends—back bending, by bringing the spine into extension, decreases a kyphotic curve.

There's another dynamic that has almost the opposite effect on the shape of the lumbar spine, yet it can cause thoracic and neck issues similar to those that excessive lordosis causes in the lower back. In our new, equally pain-inducing scenario, tight hamstring muscles pull on the sit bones, tipping the pelvis backward and flattening the normal curve of the lumbar spine. And even though it's important to strengthen your abdominal core to support a natural curve in your lower back, an overly strong or tight abdominal core may also contribute to a flattened lower back.[6]

A flattened lower back doesn't have the same structural stability as a lower back in its natural curve because the muscles weaken as they flatten out. A lower back in this condition will more easily overround backward in a forward-bending position. The thoracic spine then overworks to compensate for the instability of the lumbar spine, which results, again, in the musculature tightening up and contracting while the neck and head shift forward. In another response to a flattened lower back, the entire spine can flatten out. In this case all the myofascia weakens, creating vulnerability in the vertebrae and spinal disks from the sacrum all the way up to the cervical spine.

In all these scenarios, there's imbalance and tightness throughout the spine, from the base of your lower back up to the top of your neck. These shifts can happen almost imperceptibly and over a long period of time. By the time you feel lower back or thoracic pain, the shift in your musculature has become well set, and you have significant work to do to reshape it.

Fortunately, though, muscles love to stretch and "breathe." One of the great joys of being a yoga teacher is watching a student's tight back change its shape through yoga practice. I've watched as students' upper torso and back muscles elongate and become toned. It's as if someone opened the windows into a student's chest, letting in soft breezes to slowly and gently rinse away imbalances and tension.

Anatomy of the Upper Back

Before we move ahead, and because this is an area of the body we haven't explored, let's take a brief trip through five of the major muscle groups of your upper back: the "lats," "traps," rhomboids, serratus, and erectors (illustration 18). Their tone has an important role to play in your journey into wellness:

- Latissimus dorsi: You first encountered these muscles, typically called the "lats," in chapter 4 because they straddle the thoracic and lumbar spines. They are the largest upper back muscles, and they are responsible for stabilizing the spine in back-bending and forward-bending movements, as well as adduction (moving toward the body), internal rotation (turning inward), and the extension of the shoulder joint back and away from the front of the body. The lats start at the lower thoracic spine, right above the top of your lumbar spine and at the top of the back hip bones. They wrap around and up the sides of the body, where they interact with the oblique abdominal muscles and help with spinal stability, and then they attach to the inside of your upper arm bones.[7] I'm sure I only need to mention the name of swimmer Michael Phelps, who holds the

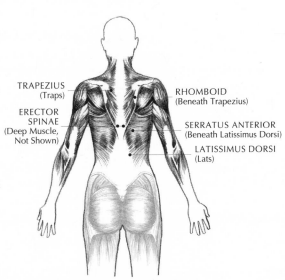

TRAPEZIUS
(Traps)

ERECTOR
SPINAE
(Deep Muscle,
Not Shown)

RHOMBOID
(Beneath Trapezius)

SERRATUS ANTERIOR
(Beneath Latissimus Dorsi)

LATISSIMUS DORSI
(Lats)

Illustration 18. The Muscles of the Upper Back

all-time record for the most Olympic gold medals, for you to visualize well-developed lats.[8]

- Trapezius: The "traps" are the large muscles that lie on either side of the upper spine, forming a large V-shape. They start at the base of your thoracic spine at T12, spread out and up along your back, and attach to your shoulder blades and the base of the skull bone at a point called the occiput. When you engage the lower traps, at your middle back, your shoulder blades are drawn down and away from your neck, an action called "depression." This simple action has a ripple effect: It elongates the neck muscles, especially in a back-bending position, which allows the head to shift into alignment over the shoulders; it encourages the shoulders to draw back, and it broadens your upper chest.

  The intermediate traps work with the rhomboids to draw the shoulder blades together, a movement called "retraction." I'd like you to feel how these two actions, depression and retraction, work together to create support for your upper chest. First, using your lower traps, "depress" your shoulder blades down and away from your neck. Find your intermediate traps by "retracting" your shoulder blades toward your spine. Now visualize your shoulder blades as "helping hands" easing your shoulders into alignment from behind and creating support for your upper chest as they gently "hug" your upper back.

  The upper traps lift the shoulder blades up. You can find your upper traps simply by lifting your shoulders up toward your ears, a movement called "elevation."

- Rhomboids: These muscles attach your spine to your shoulder blades and work with the intermediate traps to retract your shoulder blades. When poor postural habits cause the shoulder blades to slide away from the spine, the rhomboids first become overstretched and weak, and then tight and rigid. Upper back pain due to weak and tight rhomboids can be felt as chronic achiness or sharp pain along the edges of the shoulder blades.[9]

- Serratus anteriors: These muscles work reciprocally with the rhomboids—they pull the shoulder blades away from the spine. Shortened serratus muscles draw the shoulder blades out to the outer back rib cage, straining and weakening the rhomboids. When a person has both a tight serratus and strained rhomboids, it's a good bet they also have an exaggerated kyphotic thoracic spine.[10]

- Erector spinae: You also first explored this group of long, complex muscles in chapter 4 (page 130). Your "erectors" have many jobs; they bring your spine into forward bending (flexion) and back bending (extension), and, possibly most importantly, they also hold your spine in an upright position. They begin all the way down in the layers of the lower back fascia and climb up your spine, connecting with each vertebra, all the way to the base of the skull (occiput). The outer layers of the erector spinae group are long and strappy-looking—these are the muscles that become thick, short, and very prominent in a lower back with an exaggerated lordosis. They become spread out and weakened (and achy!) in an upper back with an exaggerated kyphosis. The deeper layers of the erector spinae muscles connect vertebrae to each other, forming a pattern that resembles a long braid as they weave their way up from the sacrum to the occiput.[11]

YOUR UPPER BACK IS PRIMED AND READY

Although our work so far has focused on the lower back, many of the poses you've practiced also strengthen and tone your middle and upper back musculature. So you're primed and ready for the poses to come in this chapter! Revisit the following poses for an *aha!* moment on how they recruit your middle and upper back:

- Bridge Pose, page 56
- One-Legged Bridge Pose, page 70
- Noble Warrior Pose, page 52
- Side Angle Pose, page 53
- Triangle Pose, page 69
- Table-Balance Pose, page 100
- Supported Cobra Pose, page 104
- Supported Locust Pose, page 106
- Flowing Bridge Pose, page 151
- Flying Locust Pose, page 152
- Swimming Locust Pose, page 153
- Cobra Pose Flow, page 163

Anatomy of the Neck

Not to worry, you won't be tested on all of these muscle names! But as you prepare to practice the poses in this chapter, it will be helpful to understand a little about the major muscles in your neck. The full list of muscles that allow the head and the neck to move can sound intimidating, yet when you read their names, with their repeated use of the Latin words for "long," "upright," and "head," you understand the function of these muscles—to maintain the long and upright spine we've worked on throughout this book and, of course, to support your head on top of your spine. Instead of overwhelming you with the whole kit and caboodle, I've chosen four major neck muscle groups I think you'll relate to easily (illustration 19):

- Sternocleidomastoids: Commonly abbreviated as the SCMs, these muscles are recognizable as the long, thick muscles in the outer layers of the front of the neck that run angularly up from the breastbone and collarbones to the sides of the temporal bones (the bones at the side and base of your skull). They attach to the skull right behind your ears. The SCM muscles assist with cervical and upper spine flexion, as in an abdominal crunch, in Chin Locks, which you'll practice on page 236, and with all aspects of head movement.[12] If you press your hand against your forehead and push into it with your head, you will feel your SCM muscles contract. Perhaps you've seen a person whose head is forward, whose chin is lifted, and whose back neck is shortened . . . perhaps you've experienced this postural misalignment yourself. This is the very challenging result of tightness in the SCM muscles.[13]

- Scalenes: This muscle group is actually three pairs of muscles in the sides of the neck. They originate from cervical vertebrae C2 to C7 and they extend down through the neck to where they attach at your first and second ribs. The scalenes are responsible for side flexion of the neck, and they lift the first and second ribs. When you tilt

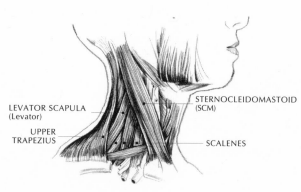

LEVATOR SCAPULA (Levator)

UPPER TRAPEZIUS

STERNOCLEIDOMASTOID (SCM)

SCALENES

Illustration 19. The Muscles of the Neck (Side View)

YOGA FOR A HEALTHY LOWER BACK

your head back and flex your neck toward your right shoulder, you will feel your left scalenes stretching.[14]

- Levator scapulae: The "levators" run along the back and sides of the neck from cervical vertebrae C1 to C4 down to the inner upper edges of the shoulder blades, the place where tension commonly settles into the upper back. You can easily find this point by swinging one arm around the front of your chest to the opposite shoulder as if patting yourself on

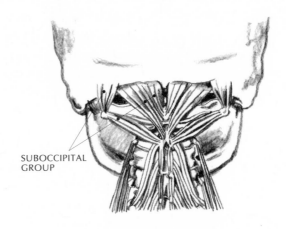

SUBOCCIPITAL GROUP

Illustration 20. The Muscles of the Neck (Back View)

the back. Your fingers will land on or very near the inner upper edge of the shoulder blade. Shift your fingers slightly toward your spine and you'll find the spot. You're feeling the traps, with the levators underneath. If you massage them, you may feel some tenderness there . . . and maybe you'll release some tension in the process! Just as their name sounds, their main function is to elevate (lift) your shoulder blades.[15]

Tightness and shortness in the scalenes and levators are usually caused by the subtle tensions that slip deep into the shoulders over time, whether from hunching over a computer, slouching against the wind on a cold winter's day, or struggling with underlying life pressures and stress. Trauma or injury can cause a startle response that shortens the musculature of the front of the body and pulls the shoulders up toward the ears and forward, creating the same tightness and shortness in these muscles. Stretching the muscles with yoga postures will help to release tension and drop the shoulders away from the ears.

- Suboccipital group: This is a group of short, deep muscles that connect the back base of the skull to the top of the cervical spine (illustration 20). Sometimes it's called the suboccipital "star," which is exactly what the muscles look like when viewed from behind. They radiate up and out to the base of the skull from the star's center at cervical vertebrae C1 and C2. The suboccipitals, as well as the scalenes, are limited in their movement and can prevent the SCMs from releasing tension, because they may reach their limitation long before the superficial SCM is brought into a stretch.[16] To find your suboccipitals, massage the "valleys" just below the base of your skull at the back with your thumbs until your thumbs go beyond the outer layers of muscles and find the deeper muscles under the occipital ridge (the bottom edge of the occipital bone). Now, here's an amazing feeling: Keeping your head still, move your eyes right and left and up and down, and you will feel your suboccipitals move. According to Thomas W. Myers in his book *Anatomy Trains*, these muscular and eye movements are so fundamentally connected that any eye movement will produce a change in tone in the suboccipitals. From there, "the rest of the spinal muscles 'listen' to the suboccipitals and tend to organize by following their lead." Myers literally means "the rest of the spinal muscles"—all of them. He says, "Loosening the neck is often key to intransigent problems between the shoulder blades, in the lower back, and even in the hips."[17]

Congratulations! Physically speaking, you've traveled the full length of your spine. You have a good understanding of the nature of your spine and how all its parts work together. Well, maybe you don't think the parts of your spine "work together" *yet,* but they will as you create tone and fluidity within your back body. Your spine, and especially your lower back, will thank you for all the time you invest in your journey into wellness.

A "HEAD START" ON YOGA FOR YOUR NECK

You may not know it, but all the spinal twists we've practiced so far in this book have been gently elongating the sides of your neck. These are good base poses to help undo tightness in the SCMs, scalenes, upper trapezius, and levator scapulae muscles, and I encourage you to continue to practice them alongside the new poses you'll learn:

- Restorative Twist Pose, page 111
- Chair-Seated Twist, page 114
- Reclining Spinal Twist, page 141
- Marichi's Seated Twist, page 158

Through Eastern Eyes: The Energetic View

Now you'll explore the middle back, upper back, and neck from an energetic perspective, which really means discussing the four upper chakras, from your heart to the crown of your head (illustration 21). They are:

- **Anahata chakra:** The fourth chakra is your heart center, located in your upper chest. Commentaries on the Yoga Sutras of Patanjali refer to the heart chakra as the "seat of intelligence"[18] and the "seat of pure knowledge."[19]
- **Vishuddha chakra:** The throat is the home of the fifth chakra, which is also considered to be the seat of pure sound in the body and the "great doorway to liberation."[20]
- **Ajna chakra:** The brow, or the area known as the "third eye," is where the sixth chakra resides. It is believed to be the seat of meditation in the body; in it, "the mind reaches a state of undifferentiated cosmic awareness."[21]
- **Sahasrara chakra:** The seventh and final chakra is called the "crown chakra" because it is found at the very apex of the body. *Sahasrara* means "thousand-spoked," and it is often depicted as a thousand-petaled lotus that sits at the crown of the head.[22] It is a powerful place of freedom from ego; deep, cosmic self-actualization; and "the seat of the self-luminous soul."[23]

The fourth and fifth chakras are the most germane to our work in the middle back, upper back, and neck, so we'll explore them more now.

Recall and visualize Kundalini, your coiled spiritual energy, and imagine it snaking its way up the energetic channels (nadis) in your spine, starting from your lower sacrum. So far, we have imagined how Kundalini energizes the Muladhara (root) chakra, the Svadhisthana (sacral) chakra, and the Manipura (navel) chakra. We have envisioned it untying the Brahma granthi, the energetic knot at your navel,

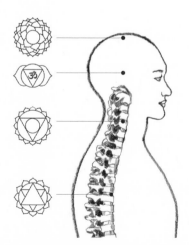

SAHASRARA
(Crown)

AJNA
(Third Eye)

VISHUDDHA
(Throat)

ANAHATA
(Heart)

Illustration 21. The Anahata, Vishuddha, Ajna, and Sahasrara Chakras

and igniting the powerful fire of transformation—agni—in your solar plexus. Now, as you open and tone your middle and upper back, visualize Kundalini continuing its upward journey into the spaciousness of your chest.

Its next stop is the Anahata chakra, situated right in the middle of your chest. I introduced you to the Anahata chakra on page 35 as the place where the energies of your lower body (apana vayu) and your upper body (prana vayu) unite. Now we'll go deeper into understanding Anahata's role in your body, both physically and energetically.

Anahata Chakra: Your Heart Center

Anahata chakra is Sanskrit for "wheel of unstruck sound."[24] In yogic philosophy, the Anahata chakra is where the silent, cosmic vibration of OM, the seed of all sounds, can be heard as one draws inward into a state of meditation.[25] It's also the place where intelligence, of both the mind and the heart, reside and merge.[26]

The Anahata chakra aids the functions of the lungs and heart by feeding them with prana, life force. The Ayurvedic marma points on the chest, called *Hrid marmani,* or heart points, help regulate cardiac function and heart rate, improve coronary circulation, and help to maintain optimal function of the lungs.[27]

When I visualize Kundalini energy rising up out of the Manipura chakra into the Anahata chakra, I imagine it as if the energy were bursting out of fire into cool, fresh air. This should be even easier to visualize when I tell you that the Anahata chakra is the home of the element of air in your body, the place of akasha (radiance, luminous inner space) and prakasha (luminosity, brightness).[28]

The Anahata chakra is also called "the seat of balance" in the body. It sits in the center of the body, with three chakras below it and three above it; it circulates air and energy through the body in all directions to balance the flow of prana; and in Indian theology it harmonizes the energy of Shiva, the "male" energetic principle of consciousness, with Shakti, the "female" energetic principle of action.[29]

I introduced the concept of the three energetic knots called granthis on page 177. You may remember that *granthi* is translated as a "knot," "hardening," or "complaint," and that Brahma granthi is the knot in the Manipura (navel) chakra.

Another knot is the Vishnu granthi, which is located in the Anahata chakra. Although I don't feel thrilled when I think about a knot in my heart, I've always liked that Vishnu granthi is so named. In Hindu mythology, Vishnu is the manifestation of universal energy charged with preserving the cosmos, and your heart is the center of your own preservation, both physically and energetically. Vishnu granthi is the knot that hardens as our emotions and emotional attachments develop, and you may gain great inner peace if you untangle it. The pranayama practice Bellows Breath (page 183) opens the granthis—and all the chest and upper back openers in this chapter may help to keep the Vishnu granthi from reknotting itself.

Vishuddha Chakra: Your Inner Voice

As you practice some of the poses that help your neck to release, you'll also open the energetic pathways leading into the throat, allowing the Vishuddha (throat) chakra to become open and active. The Vishuddha chakra, which means "wheel of purity," is the seat of self-expression and communication in the body.[30] If you've ever gotten "all choked up" with emotion, you know what the Vishuddha chakra is all about. When you speak the truth and you know that your self-expression is authentic, sincere, and pure— spoken with a clear, strong voice—this is also the Vishuddha chakra. In yogic philosophy, all spoken language comes from the throat chakra, giving voice to the emotions in the heart. When your throat chakra is open, your voice penetrates "to the heart of the listener," as one Indian author and teacher puts it. "This pure sound affects the listener by changing the space of his mind and being."[31]

In certain yogic traditions, the Vishuddha chakra is considered to be a "*stupa*,"[32] or summit, within the body. The two chakras above Vishuddha— the Ajna (third eye) chakra and the Sahasrara (crown) chakra—are considered to be in the realm of "ether," so Vishuddha is the place in the body where the four classical elements of earth, water, fire, and air (represented by the chakras below it), meet and are synthesized:

- The earthiness of the Muladhara (root) chakra
- The fluidity of the Svadhisthana (sacral) chakra
- The fieriness of the Manipura (solar) chakra
- The airiness of the Anahata (heart) chakra

Drawing together with the ethereal qualities of the top two chakras, these elements are all refined into their purest essences in the throat chakra, dissolving into pure energetic akasha, or radiance.[33]

Uniting East and West: The Holistic View

Before we begin our final sequence of new yoga poses, I'd like to take you through a meditation on your upper body and the ways in which it, like your pelvic bowl, is a vessel of energy and power in your body.

The Sanskrit word *kumbha* means "a water pot, a pitcher, a chalice."[34] In yoga practice, the word *kumbhaka,* which is derived from *kumbha,* refers to breath retention during pranayama, either when you hold your breath in at the top of an inhalation (*antara kumbhaka,* or internal retention), or when you suspend your breath at the end of an exhalation (*bahya kumbhaka,* or external retention). Patricia Walden, my yoga teacher, often refers to the human chest as a kumbha—"a sacred vessel" for holding prana (life force). For the next few minutes, I'd like you to imagine your chest in this way, as a sacred vessel for gathering and holding prana.

Sit comfortably, either on the floor or on a bolster. If your lower back is uncomfortable, sit with your back against a wall with a small pillow behind your lower back, or sit up on a chair. Drop your sit bones down into the support of your seat, while you energetically lift your torso up with a deep inhalation. Maintain the lift of your trunk as you exhale. Close your eyes and bring your attention to the back of your body.

Without arching your lower back, lift your sacral joints, back hip bones, and spinal muscles upward. Visualize them long and even on both sides of your spine. Visualize the gentle, natural curvature of your whole spine; the inward curve of your lumbar spine, the transition between inward and outward curves at your middle back, the subtle outward curve of your upper back, and the soft inward curve of your neck. Balance your head on your neck by drawing your ears in line with your shoulders while you gently tuck your chin. With each inhalation, visualize breath flowing up through your spinal muscles, supplying them with fresh oxygen and blood so they are strong and fluid.

Now you'll refine your position using what we learned about the musculature of your upper back and chest. First, draw the muscles of your upper back toward your spine—without gripping or overhardening. Visualize your lats, traps, rhomboids, and erector spinae muscles all drawing toward the center of your back. If your upper back is achy, this action should bring it some comfort. You should feel your shoulders draw back slightly and your upper chest should broaden.

Second, create the "depression" movement in your shoulder blades that I described on page 208: Draw them down from your neck toward your back waist while remaining mindful not to overarch your lower back. Hug your shoulder blades with your traps and feel the support of "helping hands" on your back. Feel that you've created a space in your chest, like the cup of a sacred chalice, to hold prana, life force.

When your back is comfortable, shift the focus of your mind from your physical body into your energetic body. Visualize your breath flowing up through the central energetic channel in your spine, the Sushumna, and through the dancing, curving channels of energy, Ida and Pingala, which weave their way up the Sushumna, meeting and crossing at each chakra. Just as you visualized energy flowing up through your spinal muscles, now visualize prana flowing up through these channels, from the Muladhara (root) chakra all the way up into the Sahasrara (crown) chakra, supplying each chakra with fresh prana so they are all open and fluid.

Now, unite your physical and energetic bodies together. Visualize your spinal muscles surrounding the Sushumna offering it physical support, while the Sushumna feeds your body energetically. Visualize Ida and Pingala dancing around and through your spinal muscles as well as around the Sushumna, embracing the muscles with nourishing energy. Visualize your physical and energetic spines completely united, physically toned, energetically spacious (akasha) and luminous (prakasha).

Come into Ocean Breath, gently constricting the back of your throat so your breath sounds like the rhythm of the ocean as it laps up onto the shore and slowly, gently flows back into its depths. Create an even, balanced rhythm to your inhalation and exhalation.

When you're ready, hold your breath for a few seconds at the top of an inhalation in the "internal retention" (antara kumbhaka) action I described earlier. Tuck your chin slightly, as if to bow your mind to your heart, and revisualize your body—especially your chest—as a kumbha, a sacred vessel for holding prana. Visualize your vibrant, plentiful prana gently diffusing itself from the kumbha of your chest into every cell of your body. Before your mind or your body becomes tense, release your holding with a long

Ocean Breath exhalation—see if the length of your exhalation can be longer than your inhalation. At the end of your exhalation, suspend your breath for a few seconds in the action I described as "external retention," or bahya kumbhaka. Repeat Ocean Breath with internal and external retention for a few rounds, as long as your mind and body remain comfortable.

Studies have shown that mindfully holding your breath and elongating your exhalation when you practice Ocean Breath can actually deepen the feeling of a calm and quiet mind.[35] Sit quietly and observe how *your* mind has changed during this meditation and pranayama practice, and reflect on the power of your breath, the kumbha of your chest, and your whole body.

Yoga Poses for a Healthy Middle Back, Upper Back, and Neck

Ask and Listen: Preparation for Practice

Passive Chest Opener

This is a supported position that stretches the pectoral muscles (your "pecs"), which run across the upper chest. When these muscles are tight, two things happen: They rotate the head of the upper arm bones forward and inward, resulting in rounded shoulders and a collapsed chest, and they pull the shoulder blades away from the centerline of the spine and forward, which causes an exaggerated kyphosis of the upper back and weakened

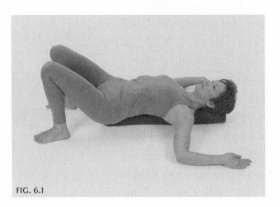

FIG. 6.1

upper back myofascia. Passive Chest Opener is particularly effective for an exaggerated kyphosis and a tight upper chest or shoulder girdle.

Open up a blanket so it's between three and four feet in length, or as long as your body is from your tailbone to the crown of your head. Roll it up tightly along the long side so it's very firm. It's important that the roll be narrow—if it's too wide, you won't feel a stretch across the front of your chest. Place the

POSES FOR YOUR OPEN CHEST

Passive Chest Opener increases broadness across the upper chest and increases the range of movement in your upper back. You'll feel how it helps in poses where your shoulders are in extension (when your arms move back and away from your body). We've done several so far, and we'll add more later in this chapter:

- Bridge Pose, page 56
- One-Legged Bridge Pose, page 70
- Open Heart and Standing Seal Variation of Deep Side Stretch Pose, page 149
- Bow Pose, page 229
- Camel Pose, page 231

roll lengthwise on your mat. Sit on one end of the roll with your feet flat on the floor and lie down on it; your entire trunk and head should be supported by the roll (fig. 6.1). A four-inch foam exercise roller is also an excellent prop for this exercise and can be used instead of a blanket.

Stretch your arms out at a ninety-degree angle from your trunk and rest them on the floor with your palms turned up to the ceiling. Draw your shoulder blades away from your ears using the lower trapezius muscles at your middle back, and press them toward your front body, feeling those "helping hands" support and broaden your chest.

Now bring your arms into "Cactus Pose" by bending your elbows and pointing your forearms and hands in the same direction as your head. Your forearms should be at a ninety-degree angle to your upper arms. Place your forearms on the floor, if possible, pressing your elbows down first, then your forearms and hands. If you want more stretch, add more height under your trunk.

Close your eyes and breathe deeply into your upper chest. Feel the layers of myofascia releasing tightness, allowing your chest to soften and broaden. Stay in the pose for five minutes, or longer if you are comfortable. To come out, turn to your side, rolling off your support, and bring yourself up to a seated position. If you have a shoulder injury, approach Passive Chest Opener with respect; it can be a surprisingly strong stretch for a "passive" pose.

Supported Upper Back Stretch

Place one block across your mat on its long edge, so it is at its "medium" height. Place another block about six inches behind it on its short end, at "high" height. Sit on your mat with your knees bent and your feet flat on the floor, reach back with your hands and hold the first block. Lay your upper back onto the block, making sure the block is underneath your shoulder blades and not your lower back. Place your head on the higher block. Hold your elbows and reach your arms over your head (fig. 6.2), or place your forearms on your forehead if you have a shoulder injury.

Check in with your body for a few breaths to make sure it's comfortable. If your lower back is uncomfortable, turn one or both of your blocks down to "low" height. If your upper back is flexible and you'd like more stretch, turn the block under your shoulder blades up to "high" height. Make sure your neck is in complete comfort, and add a blanket on top of your block for higher support. Finally, scoop your tailbone up toward your pubic bone to elongate your lower back, and stretch your legs straight down along the floor.

Let your upper back elongate along the block. Supported Upper Back Stretch helps lessen an exaggerated kyphotic thoracic spine. Visualize each vertebrae moving away from the one below it as the muscles elongate. Close your eyes and breathe deeply into your upper chest, feeling stretch and length. Remember the image of your chest as a chalice, and let your chest become a sacred vessel for holding prana.

Stay in the pose for five to ten minutes. To come out, engage your abdominal core muscles and press your hands down into the floor to help protect your spine as you lift your trunk back up into a sitting position.

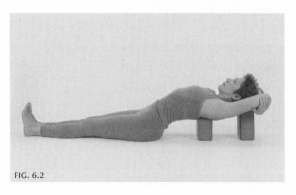

FIG. 6.2

Neck Meditation

Practice Neck Meditation often to gently release tension and increase the range of motion in your neck. If you have a neck injury, proceed slowly and with caution.

Lie on your back with your arms reaching straight out from your shoulders and your palms facing upward. Draw your shoulder blades away from your neck, press them toward your front body to open your chest and ground the tops of your shoulders. Center your head and neck on the centerline of your body and make sure that the back of your neck is long. If your shoulders are rounded upward and your head tilts back, support your head on a folded blanket. Rest your legs along the floor or bend your knees for lower back comfort.

With your next exhalation, turn your head to the right, making sure it is rotating around the axis of your spine and not tilting up or down. Your gaze should be toward your right hand. It's sometimes helpful to lift your head slightly, turn it, and then put it back down. You should be resting on your right ear. Use each exhalation to turn your head farther. Be an observer in this meditation and find out what the range of motion is in your neck. Inhaling, bring your head back to center, and repeat to the left. You might find a surprising difference from side to side!

Bring your head back to center and stay there for a few breaths; give your neck time to receive the gentle stretch of Neck Meditation.

Practice for a Healthy Middle Back, Upper Back, and Neck

Seated Neck-Stretch Sequence

Stretch

This sequence of neck stretches will gently but actively stretch the neck musculature that I outlined earlier in the chapter so that when you move into yoga poses, your neck will be a little looser and more comfortable. These aren't yoga poses per se, but their movements are incorporated into many poses. Approach them as you would any yoga practice—with mindful attention, deep and conscious breathing, and self-awareness. An extra measure of caution is appropriate if your neck is tight or if you have an injury.

Active neck stretches can be intense. Hold each stretch for only a few breaths in the beginning. Proceed slowly into deeper stretching. Most of the stretches use gentle pressure of your hands to deepen the stretch. You may choose not to do this if the stretch feels too strong; in that case simply touching your fingertips to your skull can feel stabilizing for your neck and head.

Side Neck Stretch

You'll need a chair, and a folded blanket if you like to sit on height for more support to your lower back. Sit in cross-legged position on your mat or blanket. Place the chair to your right, about eighteen inches from your body, and make sure the chair is on your mat so it doesn't slide when you're in the stretch. Hold the bottom rung of the chair with your right hand.

Lean to your left until your right arm is straight, almost to the point of being taut. Tilt your left ear down toward your left shoulder (without raising either of your shoulders) and make sure you're not rotating your head (fig. 6.3). Your eyes should gaze straight forward. Breathe into the right side of your neck and feel a good stretch—you're bringing fresh blood and energy to your upper trapezius muscles. Let your exhalations guide you farther into the stretch. For a deeper stretch, take your left hand over your head to your right ear and gently draw your head farther to the left.

Release the pressure of your hand for a few seconds, turn your eyes down to the floor, and draw your nose toward your left shoulder. Press your fingers into the back right side of your skull to go deeper into the stretch. When you feel a stretch that starts behind your right ear and goes down your neck toward your shoulder blade, you've found your levator scapulae muscle. You can gently move your head until you find the perfect stretch for your neck. Keep your hand lightly on your skull as you bring your head up and into alignment with your spine, then repeat to the left.

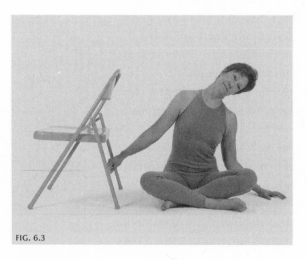

FIG. 6.3

Back Neck Stretch

Sit up tall with your head aligned with your spine. Tuck your chin slightly and draw it gently back toward your neck; you should feel the back of your neck lengthen. Exhaling, drop your chin down toward the top of your breastbone, making sure you keep your chest lifted. Move your chin more deeply with your exhalations, feeling the muscles at the back of your neck lengthen and release.

To deepen the stretch, place your fingers on the base of your skull (occiput), and press your chin farther down (fig. 6.4). You should feel a stretch to the upper trapezius muscles along the back of your neck and the tops of your shoulders. Keep your hands gently resting on the base of your skull as you lift your head back to an upright position.

Front and Side Neck Stretch

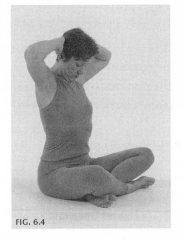

FIG. 6.4

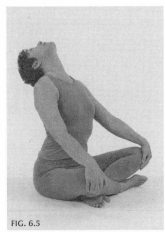

FIG. 6.5

Draw your shoulder blades away from your neck and envision those "helping hands" press them forward yet again. Place your fingers along the muscles of your neck and lengthen your neck upward. Then tip your head back, envisioning your cervical spine coming into a graceful arch. Take your head as far back as your neck comfortably allows, then slowly release your hands. Hold the base of your skull (occiput) while you tip your head back and draw it away from your neck, then release your hands and tip your head as far back as you comfortably can (fig. 6.5). Open your mouth as wide as possible to tip your head even farther back. See if you can maintain the position of your skull while you slowly close your mouth.

With your head tipped back, take your left hand to the right side of your forehead and draw your left ear toward your left shoulder. Your gaze should be upward. You should feel a stretch along the front right side of your neck at the long, thick sternocleidomastoid (SCM) muscles we discussed earlier; perhaps you can also feel a stretch to the scalenes, which sit underneath the SCMs.[36] Keeping your fingers resting on your forehead, slowly bring your head back to the center. Repeat on the opposite side.

Chair Pose

Stretch and Strengthen | Utkatasana

This pose is called Chair Pose because in it, your body looks like it's sitting in a chair. But this pose's Sanskrit name, *Utkatasana*, is translated into

English as "Fierce Pose." You'll start by opening your shoulders and side trunk, then move into a supported version of Chair Pose to warm up your back, shoulders, and chest before coming into full Chair Pose. When you practice Chair Pose after warming up, you'll feel like you are settling down into a chair that was made to fit your body, rather than moving into the fierce upper back stretch (and leg strengthener) that the Sanskrit name suggests.

Shoulder/Side Trunk Stretch

Stand about a foot from a wall, facing it. Stand farther away if your shoulders are very flexible. Draw your left arm behind your back and slowly lift your forearm and hand up along your spine until you feel a comfortable, sustainable stretch in your left shoulder. Lift your right arm up toward the ceiling and take your right hand to the nape of your neck. Crawl your right hand down your spine until your hands meet (fig. 6.6). If they don't, hold a belt with both hands.

Place your right elbow against the wall. Look to see that both sides of your chest are facing the wall evenly, and then look straight at the wall. Press your hips away from the wall and press your chest toward it as you reach your right elbow up the wall. You should feel a good stretch around the upper right trunk, shoulder, and armpit. Hold Shoulder/Side Trunk Stretch for fifteen to twenty seconds, bend your knees slightly to come out of the stretch, then repeat it to your left. If you have a shoulder injury, make sure you only go as far as your shoulder enjoys a comfortable stretch.

Supported Chair Pose

Stand facing a wall in Mountain Pose the same way you just did for Shoulder/Side Trunk Stretch, this time with your feet about eighteen inches from the wall. Lift your arms up into Upward Hand Pose. Place your hands flat on the wall, a little wider than shoulders' width apart, and stretch your arms up along the wall. Gaze straight at the wall. Bend your knees and drop your hips, coming into Supported Chair Pose.

Press your chest toward the wall while you stretch

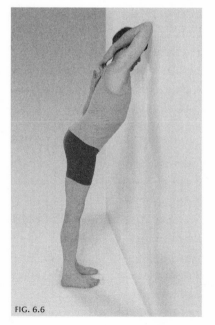

FIG. 6.6

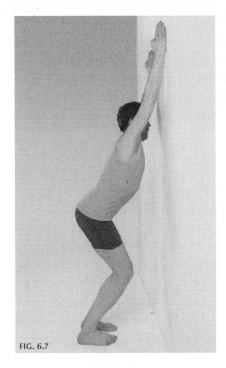

FIG. 6.7

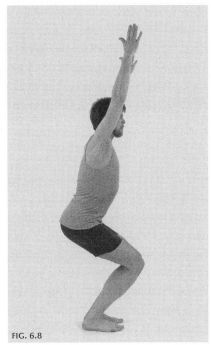

FIG. 6.8

your arms up (do not bend your elbows!), mindfully lengthening your lower back rather than overarching it (fig. 6.7). Bring your chest to the wall before your head, then touch your nose—not your forehead—to the wall. You should feel a stretch all around your upper back and shoulders, and across your upper chest. Hold for fifteen to twenty seconds, stretch your legs straight, and release the pose.

Full Chair Pose

Begin in Upward Hand Pose, this time with your palms facing each other. Elongate your body upward as you inhale, and with an exhalation bend your knees, drop your hips, and lean slightly forward (fig. 6.8). Your eyes should gaze straight ahead. Scoop your tailbone in and up to maintain length in your lower back, and stretch upward through your trunk, shoulders, and arms. Re-create the actions you found in your upper back, chest, and armpits when you practiced steps 1 and 2.

Are you able to connect with the feeling of fierceness of Full Chair Pose now? In the pose, your thighs, hips, and abdominal core musculature should be completely engaged to help your upper back open as much as possible. Hold Full Chair Pose for ten to twenty seconds, breathing evenly and fully. To come out of the pose, stretch your arms, trunk, and legs upward, come back into Upward Hand Pose, and release your arms. Stand in Mountain Pose for a few breaths and feel spaciousness and openness in your upper back and shoulders.

Eagle Pose

Balance and Strengthen | Garudasana

Stand in Mountain Pose. Stretch your arms straight out from your shoulders and as you exhale, cross your right arm over your left arm at your elbows. Face your inner forearms away from each other, and place your left fingers on the palm of your right hand. Your thumbs should point toward your face. If your hands don't reach each other, hold a belt to connect them. If you can't cross your elbows, give yourself a hug by holding each shoulder with the opposite hand. If your elbows are crossed, gaze between your forearms.

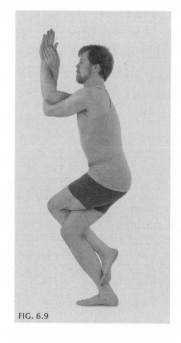

FIG. 6.9

Lift your arms upward from the elbows, and breathe into the tops of your shoulders and upper back. Feel your shoulder blades wrapping around to the sides of your trunk and feel a great stretch deep in the weave of your upper trapezius and rhomboid muscles.

You're halfway into Eagle Pose. You can remain here and just enjoy the stretch to your upper back. But if you're game to practice full Eagle Pose, you'll also get some nice openness across your sacral band. Here's the rest of the pose:

Bend your knees, just like you did in Chair Pose. Shift your weight onto your right foot and walk your left foot forward and around your right leg. Pick up your left foot and wrap it behind your outer right shin—any amount possible (fig. 6.9). This action comes from rolling your upper thighs inward, which brings your hips into internal rotation and spreads the sacral band.

Stay in Eagle Pose for fifteen to twenty seconds, mindfully

observing how your body is continually finding its balance. Consider the sharpness of an eagle's movements and intelligence, and bring those qualities into your body and mind. To come out of Eagle Pose, first undo your legs and then follow with your arms. Repeat to the opposite side.

Revolved Lunge Pose

Stretch | Parivrtta Anjaneyasana

Begin in Low Lunge Pose (page 51) with your right leg forward. Exhaling, place your left hand on the floor about twelve inches to the left of your right foot. If you can't easily reach the floor, place your hand on a block. Place your right hand on your right hip and as you inhale, elongate your trunk away from your hips. Exhaling, turn your trunk up toward the ceiling, any amount possible. Repeat the steps of elongating and turning your trunk along with the rhythm of your breath. When you've reached a comfortable, sustainable stretch, reach your right arm up toward the ceiling. To stretch your neck, rotate your head around the axis of your spine, just like you did in the Neck Meditation on page 220. Gaze forward, or look up at your raised hand for more stretch in your neck (fig. 6.10).

Revolved Lunge Pose stretches and tones the muscles of your trunk and hips. It's more important to elongate your trunk than it is to turn it, because in order to protect the spinal disks, the spine needs to lengthen before it twists. As you take your right arm up to the ceiling, be sure to draw your shoulders away from your neck and press your shoulder blades forward to help support your upper chest.

Hold Revolved Lunge Pose for fifteen to twenty seconds and slowly bring your right arm down. Place both hands on the floor and take your right leg back to meet your left leg. Rest in Child's Pose (page 61) for a few breaths before you practice Revolved Lunge Pose to your left.

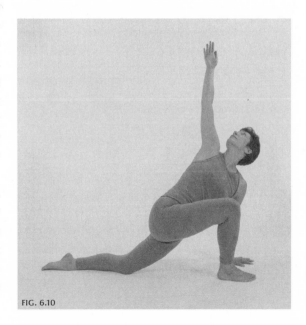

FIG. 6.10

Revolved Triangle Pose

Stretch and Strengthen | Parivrtta Trikonasana

Revolved Triangle Pose elongates all the myofascia of your lower, middle, and upper back, and it strengthens the stabilizing muscles of the legs and hips. You'll begin about six inches away from a wall, facing it. Walk your feet four and a half feet apart, and turn your right foot out and your left foot in. Place a block by the arch side of your right foot, or use a chair for support. Turn your torso to the right and swing your left arm up and around to the right. Bend forward at your hips, bring your left hand onto the block or chair, and place your right hand on your right hip. Turn your back into the wall. Elongate your trunk forward with each inhalation, and turn more deeply into the twist with each exhalation. Finally, lift your right arm up to the ceiling.

I explored the yogic concepts of practicing asanas with *sthira* and *sukham*—stability and comfort—in Deep Hip Meditation (page 42) way back at the beginning of our journey. For the next few breaths, explore your body in Revolved Triangle Pose and see if you can find these qualities in your body. Be sure your shoulders, neck, and head are in line with your spine—that's how you'll open your middle and upper back. When you're ready, lift your right arm up toward the ceiling and spread your upper chest. Turn your head just the way you did in Neck Meditation (page 220) and Revolved Lunge (page 227)—around the axis of your spine. Gaze forward, or, if you want more stretch in your neck, turn your head to look up toward your raised hand (fig. 6.1). Stay in the pose for ten to twenty seconds, or as long as you are comfortable. To come out of the pose, turn your trunk toward the chair and place your right hand on it. Step your left foot

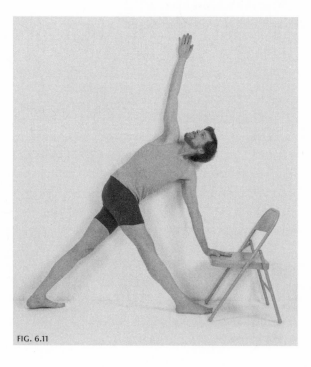

FIG. 6.11

next to your right foot, then slowly lift your trunk. Repeat the pose on the opposite side.

I often ask my students to visualize the energy of their torsos as being like a tornado when they are in this pose. It starts out narrow at its root (your hips) and it becomes bigger and broader as it twists outward (your upper chest and arms). There's nothing wimpy about this pose—let yourself fully express the power of your prana-filled vessel.

Bow Pose

Stretch and Strengthen | Dhanurasana

Now that you've warmed up your middle and upper back, check in with your lower back for a few breaths to make sure it's comfortable with the poses you've practiced so far in this chapter. If it is, you're ready to proceed into Bow Pose and Camel Pose, which are backbends that wake up and tone your entire spine. If your lower back feels tired or sore, practice the Locust Pose and Cobra Pose variations from chapters 3 and 4 until you feel confident about moving into deeper backbends.

Active Lying Down

Lie on your mat on your front body, or on a blanket for extra comfort, with your arms straight forward. You're not resting, though; press your hip bones and front groins down into the earth, and scoop your tailbone toward your pubic bone. Stretch your legs away from your waist, engage your abdominal core muscles, and elongate your trunk away from your waist. This is an active lying-down position that creates length in your lower back and helps support it in the backbend to come.

Half Bow Pose

Prop yourself up on your left forearm, bend your right knee, reach back with your right hand, and hold your foot. Press your shin and foot away from your body so your chest lifts (fig. 6.12). As it does, keep elongating your spine toward your front body, as if your spine could kiss your heart.

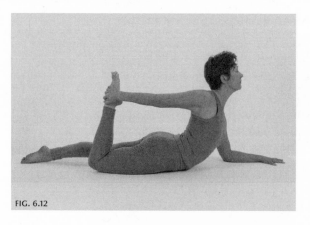

FIG. 6.12

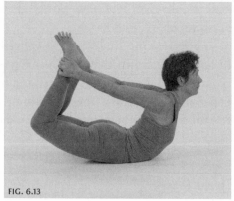

FIG. 6.13

Raise your chest only as much as your lower back comfortably allows. Hold for ten to fifteen seconds, then bring your right leg back to the floor. Place your head on your hands and rest for a few breaths, and repeat to the left.

Full Bow Pose

Once Half Bow Pose feels comfortable in your lower back, you're ready for the full pose. You'll start in step 1, "Active Lying Down" position. One at a time, bend your knees, reach back with your hands, and hold your feet (fig. 6.13). If you can't reach your feet, place a belt around your ankles and hold the belt with both hands. Draw your shoulder blades away from your ears and press them forward to broaden and support your chest.

Inhale strongly and deeply, and lift your chest and legs evenly up from the floor. Drop your chin slightly and draw your ears back, bringing your head and neck into alignment with your spine. Your eyes should gaze forward and feel soft, as if they were looking inward rather than outward. Then, if your neck is comfortable, lift your chin up, gazing softly upward. Feel your body rising up from the earth from the rootedness of your hips, your whole body curving into a smooth, curved cup shape; let your entire spine, from your tailbone to the nape of your neck, become a sacred vessel brimming with prana.

Hold Bow Pose for ten to fifteen seconds and then release your legs. Place your head on your hands, bend your knees, and lift your shins upward; gently sway them back and forth like windshield wipers for a few breaths. Rest in Forward-Bending Hero's Pose (page 107) to give your spine a few moments to stretch and release any tightness.

Camel Pose

Stretch and Strengthen | Ushtrasana

If you're game for one more backbend, practice Camel Pose. It's basically the same shape in your body as Bow Pose, but it's done in a kneeling position. This creates a little more of a challenge for the lower back, since you're leaning back to move into the pose. To protect against lower back compression, you'll first practice Camel Pose with the support of a chair so that you learn its movements in a way that brings length into your lower back.

Supported Camel Pose

Kneel on your mat with a folded blanket underneath your knees and shins for extra comfort. Place a folding chair facing you, with the seat of the chair touching the front of your hip bones. Place your hands on the side edges of the seat of the chair. Bend your elbows toward your side ribs and come onto your fingertips. Scoop your tailbone in and up and create lift in your hips and length in your lower back; engage your abdominal core muscles to create firmness in your trunk.

Press your fingertips down and lift your chest up, as if you could lift yourself all the way to the sky. This is the key to creating space and comfort in your lower back. Draw your shoulder blades away from your ears, and press them forward to create "helping hands" of support for your upper chest. Now you are supported at both the base and top of the spine, by your tailbone and your shoulder blades, respectively. Feel your chest broaden and lift as you inhale, like a wellspring of rising energy, and feel a subtle inner lift through your spine as you exhale.

Elongate the back of your skull away from your shoulders, and if your neck is comfortable, take your head back and gaze up toward the sky (fig. 6.14), softening your eyes as you did

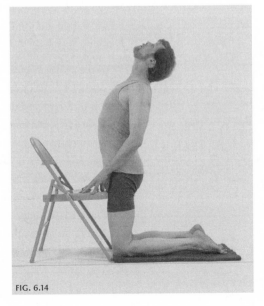

FIG. 6.14

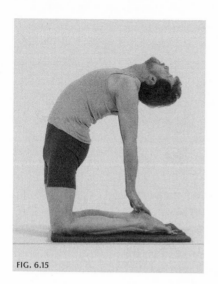

FIG. 6.15

in Bow Pose. If your neck is in discomfort, tuck your chin and gaze straight forward. To come out, release your hands, tuck your chin, and rest in Forward-Bending Hero's Pose. Check in with your lower back, and if it's comfortable, proceed into Full Camel Pose.

Full Camel Pose

Kneel on your shins and place your hands on your sacral joints. Inhaling, re-create all the supportive actions and the lift in your chest that you found in Supported Camel Pose. Draw your hands down along the back of your hips, then one by one bring your hands to your heels. Look forward, or take your head back if your neck is comfortable, visualizing that your head is cradled by supportive, loving hands (fig. 6.15). Hold Camel Pose for ten to fifteen seconds. To come out, strongly press your thighs forward to lift your chest up and back to an upright position. Rest in Forward-Bending Hero's Pose.

TIPS FOR A COMFORTABLE CAMEL POSE

Camel Pose is so strengthening for the lower back, yet sometimes it's a challenge to find a comfortable position. Here are a few suggestions to help lengthen your lumbar spine and create comfort in your lower back:

- Place a chair behind your body, with the seat of the chair touching the back of your hips, and place your hands on the chair. As the pose becomes more comfortable with repeated practice, try walking your hands down the front legs of the chair.
- Place a bolster across your calves and support your hands on it (fig. 6.16).
- Place a belt under your shins and hold it with your arms firm and stretching; lift your chest up and out of the stability of your arms.

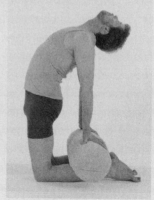

FIG. 6.16

YOGA FOR A HEALTHY LOWER BACK

Bharadvaja's Twist

Stretch | Bharadvajasana I

Your lower back will enjoy resting after backbends, but first you'll lengthen your entire spine with a seated twist to release any leftover tightness.

Sit on your mat with your legs straight in front of you. Lean to your right and shift your shins and feet over to your left hip. Place your left ankle over the arch of your right foot. Place your hands on your hips and feel how balanced they are—they should be almost even. Your left hip can be off the floor a little, but both hips should feel that they are descending down toward the earth. If you feel unbalanced, place a folded blanket under your hips. Place your hands behind you on the floor, lean back, look up, and lift your chest up any amount possible. Feel a wellspring of rising energy bubbling up your spine, just as you did in Camel Pose.

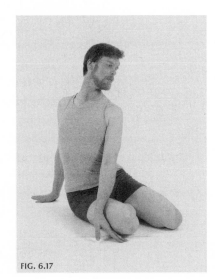

FIG. 6.17

Stretch your left arm up. With a deep exhalation, take your left hand to your right thigh. Turn your palm out and tuck your fingers underneath your thigh, stretching your palm. Press your hand against your thigh and turn your lower back, rib cage, and shoulders all to the right. Turn your neck to the right and gaze over your shoulder and toward the floor, giving the left side of your neck a good stretch. Your entire spine should be involved in the twist. For even more release in your neck, if you are comfortable, turn your head to the left and gaze beyond your left shoulder to the floor (fig. 6.17).

Hold for fifteen to twenty seconds, letting your spine deepen into the twist with each breath. Come back to center, shift your legs to your right, and twist to the left.

Child's Pose

Rest | Balasana

After Bharadvaja's Twist, come onto your hands and knees and settle your body into Child's Pose (page 61). Make sure your knees and ankles are completely comfortable so you can stay in the pose for two to three minutes, fully resting your lower back. Tuck your chin slightly and feel the back of your neck lengthen—that should feel good after you stretched it back in Camel Pose. Visualize the muscles around your neck softening and releasing. Visualize the wellspring of energy in your spine flowing freely back and forth between your sacrum and your neck in a soft wave that nurtures each nerve, disk, and vertebra along your spine.

Deep Relaxation: Find Your Inner Essence

Rest | Shavasana Variation 1

Taking the time to rest in deep relaxation after practicing backbends is as essential as practicing the backbends themselves. Lie down so that your thighs rest on a bolster, your feet rest on blocks, and your neck is supported on a rolled and folded blanket, all as shown on page 63. Before you rest, though, place your feet flat on your bolster and consider these tips to create the most comfort possible throughout your body:

- To relax your hips, gently scoop your tailbone up and press your front pelvic bones toward each other.
- To release your sacrum, draw your buttocks out to the sides of your hips.

- To elongate your lower back, draw your buttocks toward your feet.
- To elongate your middle and upper back, press your elbows into the floor and lengthen your trunk away from your hips.
- To open your chest, draw your shoulder blades away from your ears and press them toward the ceiling, then release your shoulders down into the support of the earth.
- To elongate your neck, tuck your chin slightly toward your chest, place your fingers on the base of your skull, and lengthen your head away from your shoulders.

Now let your body rest completely. You've completed the journey all the way through your spine, from your hips to your head, and through all of your chakras, from your root (Muladhara) to your crown (Sahasrara). You have found the heart of your spine—your sacrum—and your heart center—the Anahata chakra. In this relaxation you'll take a journey even deeper inward, toward "the heart of your heart," your true, essential nature.

The Yoga Sutras of Patanjali begins by stating both the goal and the result of yoga practice. Depending on which translation you read, sutra 1.2 describes yoga as "the settling of the mind into silence,"[38] "the stilling of the changing states of the mind,"[39] or "the cessation of the turnings of thought."[40] Sutra 1.3 continues by stating that, once settled, the Self "abides in its essence,"[41] "abides in its own true nature,"[42] or "stands in its true identity as observer to the world."[43] If these phrases seem lovely but esoteric to you, start by simply imagining a radiant energy that lives in your heart center. It is hidden from you by the everyday clutter of thoughts that occupy your mind. But when you take the time to quiet and still your thoughts, it shines brightly, and your resplendent, essential nature is revealed.

With these images in mind, close your eyes and draw them down into your body. Slowly travel through your body, seeing and feeling spaciousness and lightness in your hips, lower back, middle back, upper back, and neck. With your inner sight, observe your entire spine moving into complete relaxation—your muscles becoming soft and relaxed, your sacral bone and your spinal vertebrae releasing into the support of the earth.

Bring your mind to focus on your heart center, and the radiant light within it. With each exhalation, feel your thoughts becoming less important. Let go of them. Observe how your mind becomes quieter with each exhalation. After a few breaths, feel your mind remaining quiet, until the waves of thought that usually flow through you have become still. Don't worry if a thought pops back up and takes your attention away—your mind loves to think! Just let your breath carry it away and draw your mind back to your heart.

Visualize each layer of thoughts that covers the light in your heart peeling away, one by one. Let that light become more radiant and expressive until it shines completely through every part of your body, from your heart center to the farthest reaches of your fingertips and toes. Let yourself rest in the beauty of your inner light as long as you are comfortable.

When you are ready to come out, slowly move your hands and feet, roll your wrists and ankles, and bend your elbows and knees. Roll onto one side of your body and bring yourself up to a comfortable seated position. Bring your hands onto your lap. Cup your right hand over your left, then lift and join the tips of your thumbs together, forming a circle with your hands. This is one version of a hand position called Mandala mudra, which represents the intention of cultivating wholeness and calmness in oneself. *Mandala* is a Sanskrit word often translated as "circle." In the Buddhist and Hindu traditions, mantras are a kind of sacred art that symbolizes the universe and are used as an aid to meditation.[44] Sit for a few moments, honoring your body for all the work it has done in its journey into wellness and wholeness.

Grow and Progress

Chin Lock

Jalandhara Bandha

You've practiced Root Lock (Mula Bandha) to awaken the energy of your inner hips (page 39), and you've reignited your inner fire with the practice of Abdominal Lock (Uddiyana Bandha, page 191). Although you may not know it, you've also already practiced a version of Jalandhara Bandha, or Chin Lock, in the meditation we practiced in the "Uniting East and West" section of this chapter. Now we'll practice it again as preparation for a challenging—but rewarding!—sequence of poses that will bring our main work to a close.

In Jalandhara Bandha, the chin makes contact with the top of the breastbone, called the sternal notch, as a means of holding life force (prana) within the chest. You've approached this movement in Bridge Pose (page 56) and Inverted Cleanser Pose (page 155). Now that you've toned and loosened the musculature of your neck in this chapter, you'll explore Chin Lock along with Ocean Breath and internal retention (antara kumbhaka). Notice how your experience of this exercise differs from when you practiced it at the beginning of this chapter.

Sit comfortably, either on a folded blanket or in a chair. When you are ready, begin Ocean Breath (page 12). Practice between ten and twelve rounds so that both your body and your breath warm up. Feel your resonant breath flowing smoothly through your chest, and be sure that your inhalations and exhalations are even and balanced.

Now come into Chin Lock: Hold your breath in at the top of an inhalation. Lift your sternal notch up toward your chin and draw your chin down toward that spot, just below your throat. To help your chin come down,

WORKING UP TO WHEEL POSE

The following sequence will prepare your body to move into the final and most challenging new pose in this book. Wheel Pose (Upward Bow) is a deep, elegant, and invigorating backbend that awakens your entire spine in a way that celebrates all the work you've done on our journey together. Your lower back may be comfortable enough with backbends to practice Wheel Pose already, but if you got nervous just reading this, think about it as a pose that will be available to you sometime in the future. How deeply your journey into wellness takes you toward Wheel Pose depends on your particular body, your lower back health, and your intuition. Above all, listen to your body and respond to its guidance about how far it can comfortably go. If your body gives you the green light . . . go for it! If the pose feels too daunting to you, though, practice the following sequence through Bridge Pose and then rest.

Before practicing some new poses that will tone and open your trunk, legs, and hips to get you to Wheel, warm up your body by repeating some or all of these poses from earlier in the book:

Marichi's Seated Twist, page 158
Downward-Facing Dog Pose, page 145
Triangle Pose, page 69
Half-Moon Pose, page 150
Proud Warrior Pose, page 119

elongate the back of your neck and take your chin slightly forward and toward your chest. Don't worry if your chin doesn't rest on your sternal notch; all yoga practice is a process, and eventually you will come into full Chin Lock. The most important thing is that you shouldn't feel any strain at the back of your neck.

Hold your inhalation in Chin Lock for a few seconds, but not any longer than you feel comfortable. Feel your chest broad and full—a sacred vessel holding prana that diffuses softly through your body. Slowly release your breath with an Ocean Breath, releasing Chin Lock at the end of your exhalation. Repeat the whole cycle, seeing if you can retain your inhalation a little longer so that over time your internal retention can become as long as your inhalation. Practice ten to twelve rounds in this manner, taking a break between rounds whenever you feel a need to come back to a normal breath.

Revolved Side-Angle Pose

Stretch and Strengthen | Parivrtta Parshvakonasana Variation

This pose is like Revolved Lunge, but it moves into a much deeper twist. If your lower back is challenged in twisting poses, place a chair right in front of you. Begin in Supported Deep Lunge Pose (page 101) with your right leg

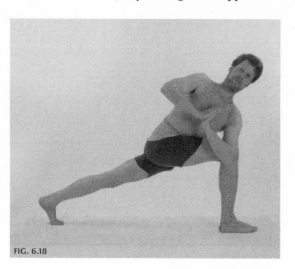

FIG. 6.18

forward and your left toes tucked under. Stretch your arms out to your sides, in line with your shoulders. Exhaling, bend from your hips and turn your trunk to the right. Bring your left arm to the outside of your right thigh.

Place your right hand on your right outer hip and check in with your lower back; if it's comfortable, take your left arm as low as possible along your thigh toward the floor, then bring your hands into Anjali mudra (page 49). Elongate your entire trunk—the front, back, and sides—as you inhale, and twist more deeply as you exhale. If your lower back is in discomfort, lift your trunk up and support your left hand on the chair. Twist only as far as your lower back comfortably allows.

Here's the fun and strengthening (and challenging!) part of the pose, which you can do regardless of how deep you twist. As you exhale, lift your left knee up off the floor while your right leg stays in lunge position. Stretch your left leg strongly from the sit bone to the heel in order to keep your leg straight (fig. 6.18). Visualize your trunk turning around your legs, the muscles of the spine lengthening from your hips all the way up to your neck. Check to see that your head, neck, and shoulders are in alignment with your spine, and press the tips of your shoulder blades forward to support and broaden your chest. Hold for ten to fifteen seconds, then bring your left knee down to the floor. Slowly unwind yourself out of the pose, then repeat to the other side.

Revolved Half-Moon Pose

Balance and Strengthen | Parivrtta Ardha Chandrasana

This is a beautiful pose that helps you develop balance as you give a deep twist to your spine and strengthen your lower back. I suggest you first practice it with your back against a wall, the same way you practiced Revolved Triangle Pose (page 228) so that you first learn to elongate your trunk and spine without worrying about balance. You'll move away from the wall as your lower back gains strength and your body becomes stable. As with the previous pose, proceed deeply into the pose only when your lower back is ready.

Begin in Revolved Triangle Pose with your left hand on either a block or a chair. Bend your right knee and step your left foot about twelve inches toward

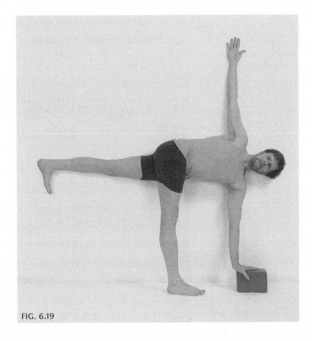

FIG. 6.19

your right foot. Walk your block forward so your left hand is under your shoulder (or walk your hand along the chair).

Inhaling, lift your left leg up until it forms a straight line with your trunk. Straighten your right leg (fig. 6.19). Breathe deeply, elongating your trunk and your left leg in opposite directions away from your hips with each inhalation, and deepen the twist with each exhalation. Be sure your head, neck, and shoulders are aligned with your spine, and gaze straight forward.

Remember the image of your trunk as a tornado, and summon the powerful, spiraling flow of energy so you can tap into and express your inner power.

To come out of the pose, bend your right knee, reach back through your left leg and place your left foot on the floor, coming back briefly into Revolved Triangle Pose. Lift your trunk up and unwind your spine. Repeat to your left.

You're almost ready to practice Wheel Pose. Before you attempt it, practice these two backbends from previous chapters in final preparation. If your body is feeling tired and Wheel Pose feels unattainable for now, end your sequence at Bridge Pose and proceed to the poses that follow Wheel Pose, before you rest in deep relaxation.

- Supported Upper Back Stretch, page 220
- Bridge Pose, page 56

Wheel (Upward Bow) Pose

Balance, Stretch, and Strengthen | Urdhva Dhanurasana

To practice Wheel Pose, it's important that you are very familiar with the instructions for Bridge Pose on page 56 because the actions of Bridge Pose create both maximum support and length in your lower back. Caution with both Bridge and Wheel Poses is advised in the presence of spinal stenosis, herniated disks, spondylolisthesis, other spinal conditions, and some shoulder injuries.

Come into Bridge Pose. Place your hands by your ears, palms down, with your fingers pointed toward your feet. Ground your feet and hands into the earth. Firm your legs and hips, scoop your tailbone up toward the sky to elongate your lower back, and engage your abdominal core muscles. Remember that the sacrum comes naturally into nutation in a backbend—it tips forward toward your front body relative to your hips and lumbar spine. Your job is to avoid excessive nutation, though. To do this, make sure that your whole spine lengthens and lifts toward your front body and that your abdominal core stays firm. Finally, create "helping hands" out of your shoulder blades, as we have throughout this chapter, to

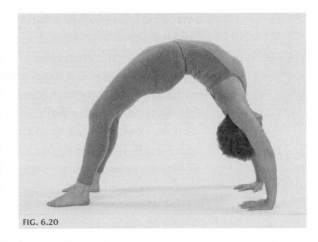

FIG. 6.20

support and broaden your chest. Inhaling, lift your hips, stretch your arms straight, and lift your lower, middle, and upper back up any amount possible (fig. 6.20).

Lift is the operative word here—everything in your body except your hands and feet should elevate so you create an even arc, a curved and unbroken channel of energy along your whole spine rather than an intense, focused bend in your lower back. You may remember back in chapter 3 that I talked about your sacrum as the keystone of the bridge your hips form as they distribute weight from your trunk to your legs. Keep this in mind as you practice Wheel Pose—the keystone of the arch is not your lumbar spine, it's your sacrum, the heart of your spine.

Visualize your spine as a luminous, graceful rainbow, each vertebra a vibrant pearl connected by Sushumna, Ida, and Pingala, the energetic channels of the spine.

Let your head release toward the floor so that your neck is long and comfortable, and gaze straight ahead. Hold Wheel Pose for five to ten seconds when you first start practicing it; slowly increase the time as you feel stronger. To come out of the pose, gently tuck your chin and lower your back body down to the floor, first onto the back of your head, then your shoulders and upper back, middle back, lower back, and hips. Make your journey out of the pose slow and gentle, maintaining the scoop of your tailbone so that your lower back elongates along the floor. Hug your knees into your chest for a few breaths and move your legs around to massage your lower back.

Wheel Pose can be a joyous experience that creates physical, mental, and emotional well-being. It lengthens tight and contracted spinal muscles, it helps to correct an exaggerated kyphotic thoracic spine, it opens the area around your heart and lungs, and it stimulates the Anahata (heart) chakra so that it's fully expansive and expressive. After practicing it, your body should feel buoyant and alive—congratulations!

When you're done practicing Bridge Pose or Wheel Pose, take time to release and relax your back. Finish your practice with two or three of the following poses to release your spinal muscles:

- Free-Your-Sacrum Pose, page 94
- Reclining Hip Twist, page 65
- Happy Baby Pose, page 93
- Restorative Twist Pose, page 111
- Decompressing Forward Bend, page 110
- Wide-Legged Standing Forward Bend, page 120
- Restorative Cleanser Pose, page 156

TIPS FOR A COMFORTABLE WHEEL POSE

Wheel Pose can be easier said than done, so here are some suggestions to help you create comfort, lift, and space in your lower back (and the rest of your body) as you practice it:

- Hold on to a partner's ankles and have your partner support your shoulder blades, literally offering the "helping hands" I've described in this chapter (fig. 6.21). This is especially helpful for opening tight shoulders and straightening the arms.
- Place the short end of two blocks against a wall with the blocks in the "low" position, about shoulders' distance apart. Place your hands on the blocks and lift up into the pose. This helps lift the middle and upper back.
- Come onto your tiptoes to lift your hips as much as possible, then lower your heels while you maintain the height in your hips.
- Belt your thighs or hips to help protect a tender lower back (see Bridge Pose instructions, page 56).

- Try a standing version of Wheel Pose: Stand about three feet away from a wall in Mountain Pose, with your back facing the wall and your feet hips' width apart. With a deep inhalation stretch your arms up over your head and as you exhale, bend your knees slightly and reach your hands back to the wall. Press your feet down strongly, engage your leg, hip, and abdominal core musculature to protect your lower back, and lift your chest as high as possible. Feel your middle and upper back arching back into a beautiful bow. Inhaling, reach your arms back up to the ceiling and bring yourself back to Mountain Pose.

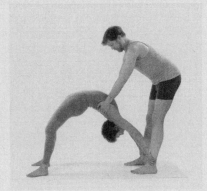

FIG. 6.21

Child's Pose and Deep Relaxation

Rest | Balasana and Shavasana Variation 1

You're now ready for a luscious, soft, restful Child's Pose! Make yourself completely comfortable, using any supports that help you completely relax your entire body (see page 62 for ideas). Once you're settled, visualize your whole spine—each vertebra, from the base of your sacrum to top of your cervical spine, and all the surrounding musculature and myofascia—surrendering into your supports and into the earth. Visualize Ida, Pingala, and Sushumna, the channels of energy that surround your spine, as completely open, and see if you can sense awakened Kundalini energy gracefully flowing through those channels, enlivening and nourishing each cell of your spine.

When you're ready to come out of soothing Child's Pose, rest completely in the deep relaxation described on page 234.

7

Maintaining a Healthy Lower Back

We have journeyed together through your entire back body, and you now have a lot of tools and resources for releasing and quieting pain in your lower back. Hopefully you have discovered new sources of strength, flexibility, and balance in your body. But your journey doesn't stop here! You are now ready to maintain your healthy lower back in ways that will keep your practice fresh and relevant to the realities of your life . . . without consuming too much of your time.

There are a number of reasons your lower back might start to slip into old patterns of pain and tension. Some of the biggies are becoming emotionally stressed, physically exhausted, or overly sedentary, spending too much time in front of a computer, or overexerting yourself in ways that can tweak an old injury or flare a condition.

When you notice any of these things in your life, don't despair that you've undermined or undone all the progress you've made toward a healthy lower back. Instead, use the same technique you use when you notice your thoughts wandering or spiraling during a meditation practice—simply give yourself a gentle reminder to come back to your center.

To help, I've drawn from the poses you learned in this book to create sequences for the five common scenarios I described above. These can supplement your regular yoga practice, or take its place if the day calls for it.

Experiment with these sequences to see how the poses might feel different from when you practiced them with your attention on a particular area of your back. Can you use your yoga to bring health and vitality to your emotional body in a time of stress, or to release a tense day of computer work, or recover from a physically taxing experience? Once you find out what works best for you in these situations, you can let go of the anxieties and self-doubt that often accompany anything that feels like a "setback."

During your practice, rest in Child's Pose at any time when your back feels fatigued. Be sure to rest in Deep Relaxation for three to five minutes at the end of any practice.

Calming Sequence for Stress

Stress is the great scourge of modern life, and you can't help but experience its reality in your day-to-day. But you know the difference between a "normal" stress level and when stress starts to take on a life of its own, building in your body and sabotaging your healthy habits. The following calming sequence can help it.

In this sequence, you will release muscle tension in your neck, upper back, shoulders, lower back, and hips—some of stress's favorite gathering places in the body. Breath practices, especially Ocean Breath with an elongated exhalation, will start to restore balance to your nervous system, calming your mind as your body starts to let go. These poses use gentle movement to counter the sharpness of stress and anxiety. See if you can find a quiet, inward focus in this sequence, letting go of agitation and an overactive mind.

1. Passive Chest Opener (a) or Supported Upper Back Stretch with Three-Part Breath (b)
2. Reclining Bound Angle Pose with Ocean Breath, breath retention, and elongated exhalation
3. Neck Meditation (see p. 220)

4. Sacral Circles (see p. 92)
5. Reclining Hip Twist
6. Big Hip Circles
7. Cow-Pose (a) and Child's-Pose (b) Flow
8. Downward-Facing Dog Pose (a), or Extended Puppy Pose (b) and Side Puppy Pose
9. Eagle Pose
10. Standing Forward Bend
11. Restorative Twist Pose
12. Restorative Cleanser Pose

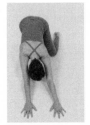
1A (FIG. 6.1)

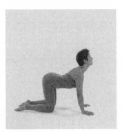
1B (FIG. 6.2)

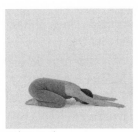
2 (FIG. 2.17)

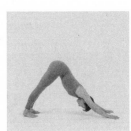
5 (FIG. 2.21)

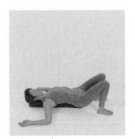
6 (FIG. 2.4)

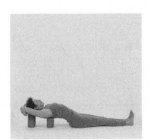
7A (FIG. 2.3)

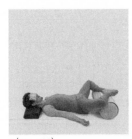
7B (FIG. 2.18)

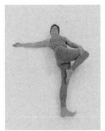
8A (FIG. 4.6)

Maintaining a Healthy Lower Back

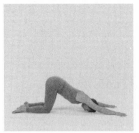 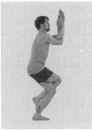 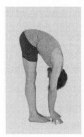

8B (FIG. 4.5)   9 (FIG. 6.9)   10 (FIG. 3.20)

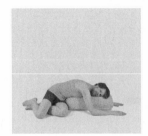 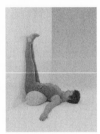

11 (FIG. 3.22)   12 (FIG. 4.16)

Activating Sequence for Fatigue

Sometimes you don't need to calm down, you need to wake up! Fatigue can be just as sabotaging to a healthy body as stress, and these poses are meant to bring mindful, prana-filled activity back into your body and mind. You will start with three breath practices to rekindle and rebuild your energy. Gentle stretches will reawaken your sacrum, hips, and lower back, opening them so that blood and energy can flow easily again, replenishing your whole body. Finally, strengthening poses will remind your body of its stamina and power, encouraging it to reconnect with its tremendous stores of energy and vitality.

1. Fire Meditation (see p. 179)
2. Shining-Skull Breath (see p. 182)
3. Bellows Breath (see p. 183)
4. Free-Your-Sacrum Pose (see p. 94)

5. Reclining Hand-to-Foot Pose
6. Reclining Spinal Twist
7. Seated Lower-Back Side Stretch
8. Revolved Wide-Legged Seated Pose
9. Noble Warrior Pose
10. Half-Moon Pose
11. Flying Locust Pose
12. Reclining Bolster Twist

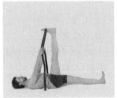
5 (FIG. 3.8)

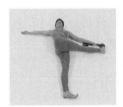
6 (FIG. 4.3)

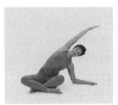
7 (FIG. 4.4)

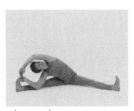
8 (FIG. 4.19)

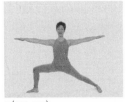
9 (FIG. 2.11)

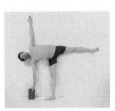
10 (FIG. 4.11)

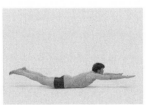
11 (FIG. 4.13)

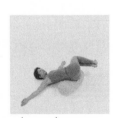
12 (FIG. 4.14)

Maintaining a Healthy Lower Back

Stretching Sequence for a Sedentary Day

Have you ever had one of those days when you realized you didn't do much moving? We all have. Maybe you were nursing a cold or other illness and were sacked out on the couch. Maybe you were behind the wheel all day, carpooling, errand-running . . . but mainly sitting in traffic. Or maybe you got absorbed in a work project and became a little too closely bound to your desk chair.

After a sedentary day, resist the temptation to dive into big movements—you could injure your stiff, tired joints and muscles. Instead, try the following poses to reawaken and reactivate your musculature—especially that of your hips and lower back, which tend to tighten the most after a period of inactivity. You will find in these poses mobility for your hips, spine, and shoulders, allowing them to release their stiffness and tension. But most importantly, these poses should reenergize your body and mind, bringing them back to that place of healthy, consistent movement and activity.

1. Standing Sacral Meditation (see p. 90)
2. Extended Puppy Pose
3. Downward-Facing Dog Pose
4. Low Lunge Pose
5. Supported Deep Lunge Pose Variation
6. Proud Warrior Flow: Proud Warrior (a) to Balanced Warrior (b)
7. Alternate Arm/Leg Prone Backbend
8. Flying Locust Pose
9. Full Bow Pose
10. Flowing Bridge Pose
11. Forward-Bending Hero's Pose, Actvie Variation
12. Head-to-Knee Pose

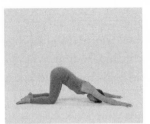

2 (FIG. 4.5)

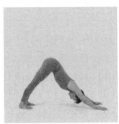

3 (FIG. 4.6)

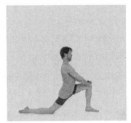

4 (FIG. 2.10)

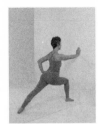

5 (FIG. 3.12)

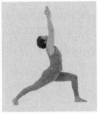

6A (FIG. 3.29)

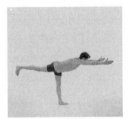

6B (FIG. 4.21)

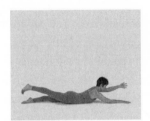

7 (FIG. 3.15)

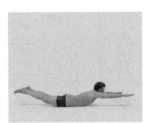

8 (FIG. 4.13)

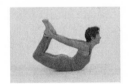

9 (FIG. 6.13)

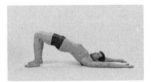

10 (FIG. 4.12)

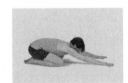

11 (FIG. 3.17)

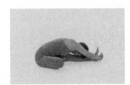

12 (FIG. 4.26)

Releasing Sequence for Computer Overuse

Computers are a fact of daily life for most of us. Even if we are using laptops or tablets, the act of sitting for prolonged periods of time with our hands outstretched, fingers tapping, has a ripple effect through the whole body, from the way the lower back can tighten and overarch in order to compensate for your forward-pulled shoulders, to the way your neck angle can tweak your sacral-joint alignment.

This sequence of poses targets your hips, lower and upper back, neck, and shoulders to release that muscle tension. It will also help you clear and refresh your mind, which can't help but be overstimulated and foggy after a lot of screen time. You can even practice most of the poses in this sequence right at your desk or in your office when it's time to take a computer break—something you should ideally do every hour. No mat required!

1. Chair-Seated Hip Opener
2. Seated Neck-Stretch Flow (steps 1–3)
3. Chair-Seated Twist
4. Standing Swan Pose
5. Standing Forward Bend Pose
6. Shoulder/Side Trunk Stretch
7. Supported Chair Pose
8. Full Chair Pose
9. Eagle Pose
10. Full Camel Pose
11. Restorative Twist Pose
12. Child's Pose

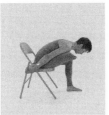

1 (FIG. 2.5)

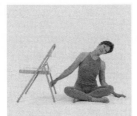

2A (FIG. 6.3)

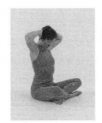

2B (FIG. 6.4)

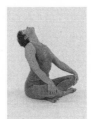

2C (FIG. 6.5)

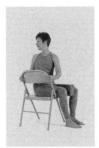

3 (FIG. 3.24)

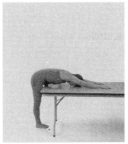

4 (FIG. 2.14)

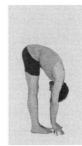

5 (FIG. 3.20)

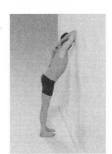

6 (FIG. 6.6)

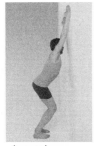

7 (FIG. 6.7)

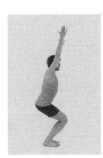

8 (FIG. 6.8)

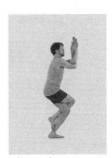

9 (FIG. 6.9)

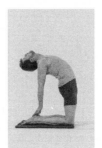

10 (FIG. 6.15)

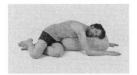

11 (FIG. 3.22)

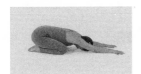

12 (FIG. 2.18)

Maintaining a Healthy Lower Back

Quieting Sequence for an Overactive Day

Shhhhh. It's time to let go of the physical and mental exertions of your day and prepare for a good night's rest. This sequence uses Ocean Breath to bring your nervous system into balance, and a series of gentle poses that rest and relax your lower back, alleviate stiffness in your hips and shoulders, and calm and quiet your mind after a full day of activity—good, bad, and in-between.

1. Reclining Bound Angle Pose with Ocean Breath
2. Reclining Sacral-Balancing Pose (steps 1 and 2)
3. Seated Crossed-Legged Pose with Variations
4. Forward-Bending Hero's Pose, Active Variation
5. Deep Hip Bend
6. Bharadvaja's Twist
7. Standing Forward Bend
8. Half Deep Side Stretch Pose
9. Flowing Bridge Pose
10. Happy Baby Pose
11. Resting Swan Pose
12. Seated Forward Bend Pose

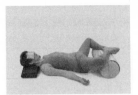

1 (FIG. 2.17)

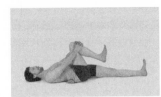

2A (FIG. 3.6)

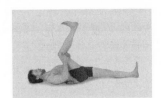

2B (FIG. 3.7)

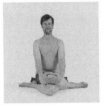

3A (FIG. 3.25)

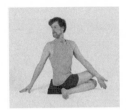

3B (FIG. 3.26)

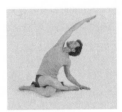

3C (FIG. 3.27)

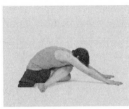

3D (FIG. 3.28)

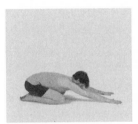

4 (FIG. 3.17)

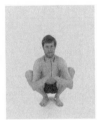

5 (FIG. 2.8)

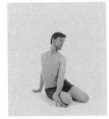

6 (FIG. 6.17)

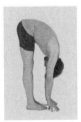

7 (FIG. 3.20)

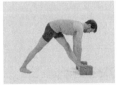

8 (FIG. 4.9)

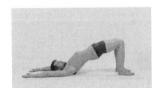

9 (FIG. 4.12)

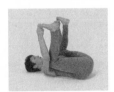

10 (FIG. 3.3)

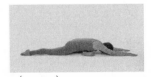

11 (FIG. 2.27)

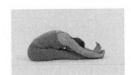

12 (FIG. 4.27)

Maintaining a Healthy Lower Back

8

PRACTICES FOR SPECIFIC
LOWER BACK CONDITIONS
AND DIAGNOSES

THE TITLE FOR THIS BOOK IS *Yoga for a Healthy Lower Back,* and I firmly believe that anyone who suffers from lower back pain can make progress toward health, if not achieve a fully functional, pain-free lower back. But for some of you, "lower back pain" has been given a more intimidating, serious name, such as spinal stenosis, spondylolisthesis, or fibromyalgia, and you may be wondering if your diagnosis means you aren't destined to be included in the "healthy lower back club."

The truth is, you may have a longer road than others whose pain is stress- or lifestyle-based. And there are some movements that are less likely to be helpful to you because of your condition. However, yoga is absolutely available to you as a tool for bringing wellness, energy, and renewed strength to your lower back—and your whole body—regardless of your diagnosis.

This chapter offers condition-specific yoga sequences, using poses we've practiced in the book, for lower back issues ranging from sacral sprain to arthritis to pregnancy. So take a look (you may even want to bring this chapter to your next doctor's appointment), take a deep breath, and see how your lower back can find its path toward health.

Practice for a Sacral Sprain

A diagnosis of "sacral sprain" means that you have injured either your hip muscles or your sacral ligaments. Sacral sprain often feels like a dull ache, and it can result in muscle spasm and painful tightness if not tended to. This sequence of poses will help relieve the pressure and pain of sacral sprain, giving the injury the chance to heal.

1. Extended Puppy Pose and Side Puppy Pose
   - Broadens and elongates your sacrum to release tightness and tension
   - Stretches your entire spinal musculature

2. Seated Crossed-Legged Pose Flow
   - The hip rotator (piriformis) and buttock (gluteus maximus) muscles are stretched and elongated to help release tension and tightness in your hips and sacrum
   - The back hips and the sacral joints are broadened
   - For a less intense stretch, practice Chair-Seated Hip Opener, page 46

3. Chair-Seated Twist
   - Sacral joints are stable in a seated position
   - The sacrum is gently stretched and the spinal musculature is massaged and elongated

4. Noble Warrior Pose
   - Strengthens the stabilizing muscles of your legs, hips, and spine
   - Lubricates your hip joints

5. Half Moon Pose
   - Broadens your hips
   - Elongates all the musculature of your spine and trunk, especially the side muscles

6. Low Lunge Pose
   - Broadens your sacrum and balances your sacral joints
   - Elongates the front thigh (quadriceps) and hip flexor (psoas and illiacus) muscles

7. Proud Warrior Pose
   - Lengthens all your spinal musculature
   - Practice Supported Deep Lunge Pose with Variations, page 101, for more support to your lower back

8. Half Deep Side Stretch Pose
   - Strengthens the stabilizing muscles of the legs, hips, and spine
   - Broadens your sacrum, elongates your lumbar spine

9. Alternate Arm/Leg Prone Backbend
   - Massages, tones, and strengthens all the myofascia of your sacrum, back hips, and lower back
   - Elongates thigh (quadriceps) and hip flexor (psoas) muscles to bring your pelvis into neutral hip position

10. Supported Locust Pose
   - Stabilizes and strengthens your sacrum and lumbar spine
   - Tones and lengthens your hip flexors

11. Reclining Bolster Twist
   - Gently massages your hips, sacrum, abdomen, and lower back while hips and spine are completely supported
   - Quiets the mind and releases mental tension

12. Supported Child's Pose
   - Rests your whole spine in a completely supported position
   - Calms your mind

See next page for photos.

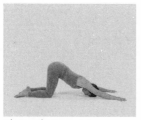 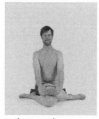 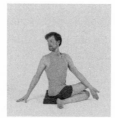 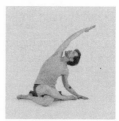

1 (FIG. 4.5)   2A (FIG. 3.25)   2B (FIG. 3.26)   2C (FIG. 3.27)

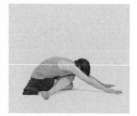 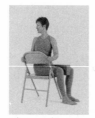 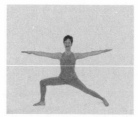 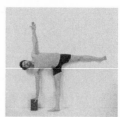

2D (FIG. 3.28)   3 (FIG. 3.24)   4 (FIG. 2.11)   5 (FIG. 4.11)

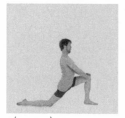 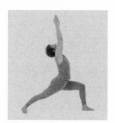 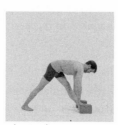 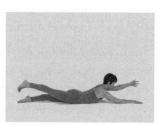

6 (FIG. 2.10)   7 (FIG. 3.29)   8 (FIG. 4.9)   9 (FIG. 3.15)

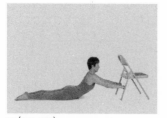 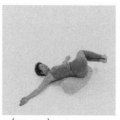 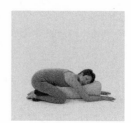

10 (FIG. 3.16)   11 (FIG. 4.14)   12 (FIG. 2.19)

Practice for Referred Sacral Pain

Referred or radiating sacral pain can be a confounding problem, because it is hard to pin down its "home base" source. The best way to treat referred pain is to offer your body gentle versions of a number of different movements, and be mindful of which ones soothe your pain, and which exacerbate it. This sequence of releasing poses will help you open your lower back body and, hopefully, break the cycle of referred or radiating pain.

1. Big Hip Circles
   - Loosens and tones your hips, sacrum, and lumbar spine
   - Massages and tones your abdominal core muscles

2. Reclining Crossed-Legged Pose
   - Stretches and elongates your hip rotator (piriformis) and buttock (gluteus maximus) muscles to release tightness and increase mobility in your hips and sacrum
   - Promotes realignment of your sacral joints

3. Partner-Assisted Leg Press
   - Promotes realignment of your sacral joints
   - Releases tension and increases mobility in your hips, sacrum, and lower back
   - Spreads your sacrum to help release tightness and compression across the sacral band
   - Practice Free-Your-Sacrum Pose if you do not have a partner

4. Reclining Hand-to-Foot Pose
   - Lengthens the hamstrings and deep hip and lumbar muscles, which increases the range of motion in your hips, sacrum, and lumbar spine
   - Helps relieve sciatic nerve pain

5. Deep Hip Bend
   - Elongates your sacral and lower spine musculature, helping compressed sacral joints
   - The supported variation at a ledge or counter creates traction and length through your entire spine

6. Standing Swan Pose (a) or Resting Swan Pose (b)
   - Stretches the buttock (gluteus maximus) muscles of your front leg
   - Stretches the hip flexor (psoas) muscle of your back leg

7. Supported Deep Lunge Pose Variation
   - Helps to realign your sacral joints
   - Stretches the hip flexor (psoas) muscle of the back leg

8. Standing Forward Bend
   - Decompressing Forward Bend, page 110, broadens and opens the sacral and lumbar myofascia, which helps to release muscular tension and relieve pressure on intervertebral disks and nerves
   - Calms and quiets your mind
   - Practice Half Forward Bend Pose, page 108, if Standing Forward Bend irritates your sacrum or lower back

9. Downward-Facing Dog Pose
   - Increases flexibility in your hips and broadens the sacral band
   - Calms and quiets your mind
   - Dangling Down-Dog Pose, page 147, is especially helpful for releasing tightness in your lower back and balancing your hips and sacrum.

10. Half Deep Side Stretch Pose
    - Stretches and tones the legs, hips, sacrum, and all spinal muscles
    - Brings flexibility to your hips and broadens the sacral band

11. Bridge Pose
    - Stretches and tones the hip flexor (psoas), abdominal, front thigh, and front chest muscles
    - Increases flexibility in your lumbar and thoracic muscles

12. Reclining Hip Twist
    - Stretches your outer hips and thighs
    - Elongates and tones your back and abdominal muscles and releases tightness in the lumbar spine
    - Opens your sacral joints

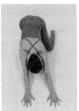

1 (FIG. 2.4)

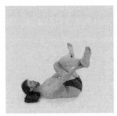

2 (FIG. 2.6)

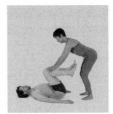

3 (FIG. 3.4)

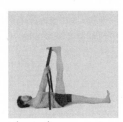

4 (FIG. 3.8)

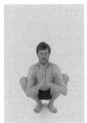

5 (FIG. 2.8)

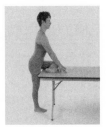

6A (FIG. 2.13)

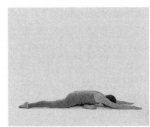

6B (FIG. 2.27)

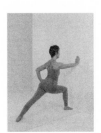

7 (FIG. 3.12)

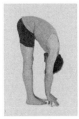

8 (FIG. 3.20)

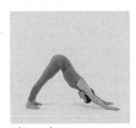

9 (FIG. 4.6)

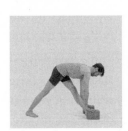

10 (FIG. 4.9)

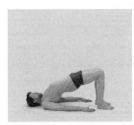

11 (FIG. 2.15)

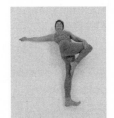

12 (FIG. 2.21)

Practice for Sacral Joint Dysfunction

Sacral joint dysfunction, also called by the name "sacral joint derangement," is usually due to an imbalance between your two sacral joints. Typically, either one side rotates forward of the other or the joints are twisted in a way that leads to uneven downward pressure into your very-low back and hips. This sequence is meant to gently open and release your sacral joints in order to bring alignment, balance, and pain relief.

1. Doorway Stand
   - Balances your pelvic bones and the sacral joints
   - Increases leg and hip flexibility

2. Sacral Circles (see p. 92)
   - Gently massages the myofascia of the sacrum
   - Releases tight sacral joints and an overarched lumbar spine

3. Free-Your-Sacrum Pose (see p. 94)
   - Spreads your sacrum to help release tightness and compression across the sacral band
   - Encourages the sides of your sacrum to ground evenly to help bring sacral joints into alignment

4. Reclining Sacral-Balancing Pose
   - Helps move a forward-rotated hip bone back into place, realigning your sacral joints as it does so
   - Brings stability to your sacral joints

5. Reclining Tree Pose
   - Strengthens the sacral myofascia and helps your sacral joints come into balance
   - Therapeutic if your sacral joints are overstretched and loose
   - Most helpful for a sacral joint that is rotated backward

6. Downward-Facing Dog Pose
   - Moving your hips in Down Dog rotates, massages, and loosens tight sacral joints, creating space for a rotated joint to move back into place

- Dangling Down-Dog Pose or working with a partner assist, page 147, balances your hips and your sacrum.

7. Proud Warrior Pose
   - Broadens the sacrum and balances your sacral joints
   - Lengthens all spinal musculature
   - Practice Supported Deep Lunge Pose with Variations, page 101, for more lower back support

8. Supported Cobra Pose
   - Draws your sacral joints toward your front body and "resets" them into a balanced position
   - Strengthens and tones the buttock (gluteus maximus), hip flexor (psoas), and the lumbar muscles.

9. Bridge Pose
   - Supporting your hips on a block is excellent for balancing the sacral joints
   - Strengthens the back hip (gluteus maximus) and lumbar and thoracic muscles

10. Happy Baby Pose
    - Spreads, elongates, and massages your sacral joints and your lumbar muscles after backbends
    - Stretches the sacral ligaments and helps to balance your sacral joints

11. Restorative Cleanser Pose
    - Rests your lower back in a gentle backbend, which helps to tone the myofascia of your sacrum and lumbar spine.

See next page for photos.

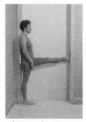 1 (FIG. 3.1)

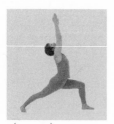 4 (FIG. 3.6)

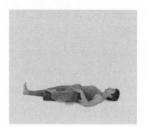 5 (FIG. 3.10)

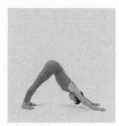 6 (FIG. 4.6)

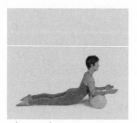 7 (FIG. 3.29)

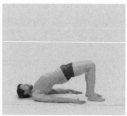 8 (FIG. 3.14)

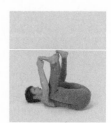 9 (FIG. 2.15)

10 (FIG. 3.3)

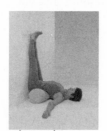 11 (FIG. 4.16)

Practice for Lordosis, Lumbar Muscular Pain, and Strain

As you learned in chapter 4, an exaggerated lordosis is a condition in which the lumbar spine overarches, straining the sacral joints, surrounding musculature, and your entire lower back body. Sometimes lordosis is a chronic condition, something you were born with; other times, it is your body's way of tightening up in times of stress. Either way, it can get in the way of progress toward a healthy lower back, so these poses will help release it and restore your lumbar spine's natural curve.

1. Pelvic Tilt
   - Massages and gently elongates the lower back muscles
   - Tones the abdominal core muscles, which counteract overarching of the lower back and supports the natural curvature of your lumbar spine

2. Cow-Pose (a) and Child's-Pose (b) Flow
   - Gently elongates your lower back in extension and massages and tones it in flexion
   - Massages your hip myofascia and abdominal organs

3. Extended Puppy Pose and Side Puppy Pose
   - Stretches and tones all the muscles of the spine
   - Helps the lumbar muscles lengthen and release tightness

4. Seated Lower Back Side Stretch
   - Targets the myofascia on the side of your trunk and lower back, especially the quadratus lumborum muscle and the iliolumbar ligament, which are often indicated in lower back pain
   - Stretching away from the "sore" side, if you have one, often provides immediate relief, especially if it feels tight or compressed

5. Table-Balance Tuck Pose
   - Elongates and massages your lower back muscles
   - Strengthens your abdominal core, which counteracts overarching of the lower back and supports the natural curvature of your lumbar spine

6. Partner-Assisted Sacrum Traction
   - Elongates the sacrum and the lumbar spine
   - Helps to decompress excessive lordosis and tight musculature
   - Practice Free-Your-Sacrum Pose (see p. 94) if you do not have a partner

7. Wide-Legged Standing Forward Bend Steps 2 and 3
   - Strengthens the stabilizing muscles of your feet, legs, and hips
   - Releases tightness and tension in your sacrum and lumbar spine

8. Flowing Bridge Pose
   - Lengthens the hip flexor (psoas) muscles, which counteracts overarching of the lumbar muscles.
   - Strengthens your hip, sacrum, and lower back muscles

9. Marichi's Seated Twist
   - Releases tightness in the spinal muscles and lengthens the entire spine, helping the vertebrae to shift into proper alignment
   - Creates upward traction in the spine, especially at the sacrum and lumbar spine

10. Standing Forward Bend Pose
    - Practice Decompressing Forward Bend with a rolled blanket between thighs and abdomen, page 110, to release tight and overarched lower back musculature
    - Gently elongates all your spinal muscles

11. Revolved Wide-Legged Seated Pose
    - Stretches and tones the quadratus lumborum muscles, as well as the erector spinae group and the latissimus dorsi muscles, which are often indicated in lower back pain
    - Stretching away from the side of your back that feels tight and painful can bring you relief

12. Head-to-Knee Pose
    - Promotes the natural curve of your lumbar spine
    - Tones the abdominal core, the legs, and the hips
    - Elongates your lower back musculature
    - Practice Seated Forward Bend Pose, page 167, if Head-to-Knee Pose irritates your sacrum, knees, or hips

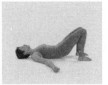 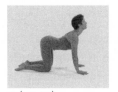 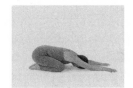 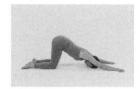

1 (FIG. 2.1)   2A (FIG. 2.3)   2B (FIG. 2.18)   3 (FIG. 4.5)

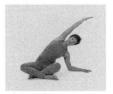 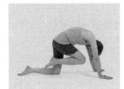 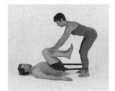 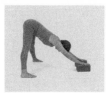

4 (FIG. 4.4)   5 (FIG. 5.1)   6 (FIG. 3.5)   7A (FIG. 3.31)

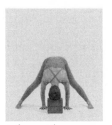 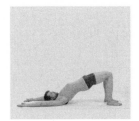 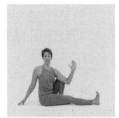 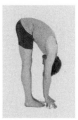

7B (FIG. 3.32)   8 (FIG. 4.12)   9 (FIG. 4.18)   10 (FIG. 3.20)

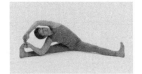 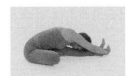

11 (FIG. 4.19)   12 (FIG. 4.26)

Practice for Herniated Disk and Pinched Nerve

Herniated spinal disks and pinched nerves are very common diagnoses, often resulting from either sudden or chronic overexertion. Spinal disks are the spongy material that cushion the vertebrae, and when those disks become overly compressed or tweaked out of alignment, they can bulge, slip, or otherwise "herniate." The injured disk often slides into a position where it puts pressure on nearby nerve endings, causing tingling, numbness, or pain down the length of your nerves.[1] These gentle poses can help support your recovery from this condition, and open your body in a way that gives your nerves room to calm down and heal.

1. Pelvic Tilt
   - Provides therapeutic, mindful rest for your lower back
   - Gently elongates your lower back musculature

2. Reclining Crescent Moon Pose
   - Provides a gentle, stretch for your lower back with your back completely supported by the floor
   - Helps release knots and scar tissue in the myofascia and strengthens the supporting ligaments of the lumbar spine on the elongated side of your body

3. Partner-Assisted Sacrum Traction
   - Elongates the sacrum and lumbar muscles, creating space for the path of nerve roots from the spine into your hips and legs
   - Opens spaces between spinal vertebrae, helping to relieve pressure on intervertebral disks and nerves

4. Reclining Sacral-Balancing Pose
   - Stretches the buttock (gluteus maximus) and elongates the lumbar musculature
   - Helps release muscle tightness and tension throughout your lower back

5. Downward-Facing Dog Pose
   - Dangling Down-Dog and its partner-assisted variations (see page 147) traction the spine and lengthen the lumbar muscula-

ture, opening the spaces between vertebrae, and help to relieve pressure on disks and nerves

- Helps to balance the spinal muscles to bring the two sides of the spine into alignment

6. Chair-Seated Twist
   - Releases tightness in the spinal muscles and lengthens the entire spine, helping the vertebrae and disks to shift into proper alignment
   - Creates traction in the spine, especially at the sacrum and lumbar areas. In the case of disk injuries, the traction can help create height at the intervertebral spaces, which brings elasticity into the disks and relief from pain

7. Full Chair Pose
   - Strengthens the lumbar muscles, which helps to support and protect nerve roots as they move through the spine[2]
   - Helps realign spinal vertebrae

8. Side Angle Pose
   - Strengthens the supporting ligaments of the lumbar on the elongated side of your body
   - Elongates the lumbar and creates flexibility along the outer hips and trunk

9. Half-Moon Pose
   - Tones and strengthens all the main movers and stabilizers of your legs, hips, and spine
   - Strengthens and elongates the lumbar musculature, helping to support and protect nerve roots as they move through the lumbar spine

10. Half Balanced Warrior Pose
    - Strengthens and tones all the spinal musculature, especially the muscles in the lumbar spine
    - Increases fluidity in your hamstrings and hips

11. Alternate Arm/Leg Prone Backbend
    - Massages, tones, and strengthens all the myofascia of your lower back while it is in a supported and stable position
    - Increases flexibility in your lower and mid back

12. Reclining Bound Angle Pose
- Provides restorative, therapeutic rest
- Resting your feet and thighs on a bolster helps to elongate your lumbar spine and allows it to rest along the ground, releasing subtle stresses and tensions

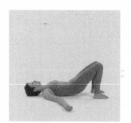

1 (FIG. 2.1)

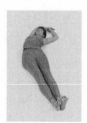

2 (FIG. 4.2)

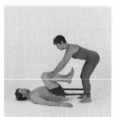

3 (FIG. 3.5)

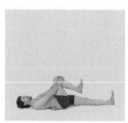

4 (FIG. 3.6)

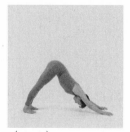

5 (FIG. 4.6)

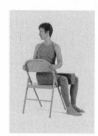

6 (FIG. 3.24)

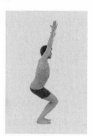

7 (FIG. 6.8)

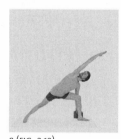

8 (FIG. 2.12)

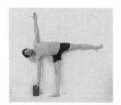

9 (FIG. 4.11)

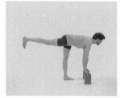

10 (FIG. 4.20)

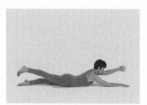

11 (FIG. 3.15)

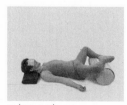

12 (FIG. 2.17)

YOGA FOR A HEALTHY LOWER BACK

Practice for Arthritis, Spinal Stenosis, and Spondylolisthesis

Arthritis, spinal stenosis, and spondylolisthesis are three conditions in which the ability of the spinal joints to move is restricted for one reason or another. In arthritis, inflammation is the culprit. Spinal stenosis is a narrowing of the spinal column, often caused by arthritis in the spine.[3] And spondylolisthesis is a condition in which lower-back vertebrae slip out of alignment in such a way that bone sits directly next to bone.[4] The goal in treating these conditions with yoga—like the sequence below—is to calm inflammation, open the joints, and encourage proper blood and fluid flow in order to allow more comfortable movement in the area.

1. Deep Relaxation Variation 1
   - Provides therapeutic, mindful rest for your lower back
   - Balances your emotions in order to help cope with chronic pain

2. Pelvic Tilt
   - Massages and gently elongates the lower back muscles
   - Increases lower back flexibility

3. Sacral Circles (see p. 92)
   - Releases tight sacral joints and an overarched lumbar spine

4. Happy Baby Pose
   - Elongates the myofascia of the lower back
   - Spreads and massages your sacral joints

5. Reclining Sacral-Balancing Pose
   - Elongates lower back myofascia
   - Creates traction for lumbar spine

6. Cat (a) / Cow (b) Cycle
   - Brings your spine into a gentle upward arch without the risk of strain or overexertion
   - Increases the disk space between the front of each vertebra
   - Provides a moment of therapeutic rest

7. Table-Balance Tuck Pose
   - Elongates and massages your lower back muscles
   - Strengthens your abdominal core, which counteracts overarching of the lower back and supports the natural curvature of your lumbar spine

8. Resting Swan Pose
   - Broadens your sacrum
   - Releases tightness in your hip and lower back muscles

9. Standing Sacral Meditation (see p. 90)
   - Gently massages, soothes, and loosens lower back myofascia
   - Increases range of motion in the lower back

10. Dangling Down-Dog Pose
    - Releases tightness in your lower back and elongates lower back musculature
    - Relieves gravitational pressure on sacral and lumbar vertebrae
    - Calms and quiets your mind

11. Decompressing Forward Bend
    - Elongates and releases tightness in all the muscles of the back body
    - Soothing and relaxing for lower back musculature

12. Child's Pose
    - Provides therapeutic rest for your spine, and quiet for your mind, both of which will help you cope with chronic pain
    - Practice with folded blankets or bolster lengthwise under your torso to completely rest your lower back

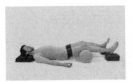

1 (FIG. 2.20)

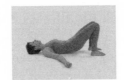

2 (FIG. 2.1)

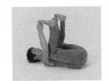

4 (FIG. 3.3)

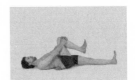

5 (FIG. 3.6)

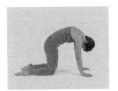

6A (FIG. 2.2)

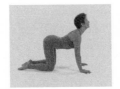

6B (FIG. 2.3)

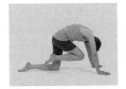

7 (FIG. 5.1)

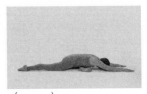

8 (FIG. 2.27)

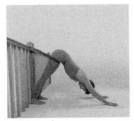

10 (FIG. 4.8)

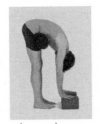

11 (FIG. 3.21)

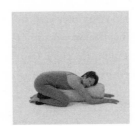

12 (FIG. 2.19)

Practice for Lower Back Health with Fibromyalgia

Fibromyalgia is a common, complex condition of unknown cause. Its main symptom is spreading pain that originates at places in the body called tender points, found in the myofascia on the back of the neck, shoulders, chest, lower back, hips, shins, elbows, and knees. Other symptoms include fatigue, poor sleep, and tiredness upon waking. It has been linked to headaches, depression, and anxiety, and it can be accompanied by irritable bowel syndrome, chronic fatigue syndrome, and restless leg syndrome,[5] as well as an overactive sympathetic nervous system.[6]

Yoga practice can be very therapeutic for fibromyalgia, as well as helping your lower back along its journey into health, when you practice very gentle movements that stretch the myofascia with complete, mindful attention to and respect for the feelings in your body. A good rule of thumb when it comes to practicing yoga with fibromyalgia is "less is more." Do not overwork your physical body, and take rest breaks often between poses using Child's Pose, Happy Baby, or Deep Relaxation.

A few hours after your yoga practice into the next day, note the feedback your body gives you and adjust your practice accordingly. If your body is sore, slow your practice down. Over time, you may find that you can increase your body's range of movement and build tone in your musculature.

The following sequence is designed to:

- Gently stretch and elongate the myofascia throughout your body with gentle and supported movement
- Balance your nervous system and calm overactive emotions using breath practice (pranayama)
- Gently build muscular tone with supported standing poses
- Provide deep relaxation and rejuvenation for your physical, mental, and emotional bodies

1. Reclining Lower Back Meditation with Ocean Breath (with elongated exhalations)

2. Reclining Bound Angle Pose

3. Supported Upper Back Stretch

4. Neck Meditation (see p. 220)

5. Sacral Circles (see p. 92)

6. Free-Your-Sacrum Pose

7. Reclining Hip Twist

8. Big Hip Circles

9. Standing Sacral Meditation

10. Triangle Pose (a, supported at a wall with your hand on a chair) or Noble Warrior Pose (b, with your hands supported on a high table)

11. Restorative Twist Pose

12. Restorative Cleanser (placing your hips and lower back flat on the floor if your back is irritated by back bending)

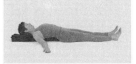

1 (FIG. 4.1)

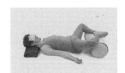

2 (FIG. 2.17)

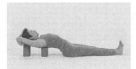

3 (FIG. 6.2)

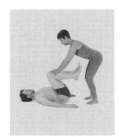

6 (FIG. 3.4)

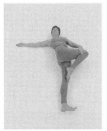

7 (FIG. 2.21)

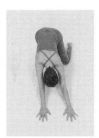

8 (FIG. 2.4)

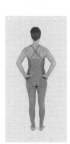

9 (FIG. 1.4)

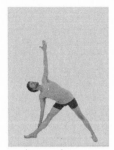 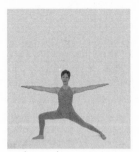 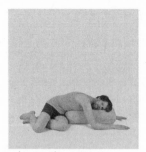 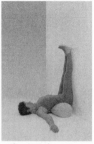

10A (FIG. 2.25)   10B (FIG. 2.11)   11 (FIG. 3.22)   12 (FIG. 4.16)

Practice for Lower Back Health during Pregnancy

As you practice yoga throughout your pregnancy, be sure to consult with a medical professional so you can meet your body's particular needs during each trimester. Most poses can be safely practiced during the first trimester in the same way you would practice them if you weren't pregnant, with caution advised against practicing abdominal and twisting poses. During the second and third trimesters, modify how deeply you go into poses, and always create space for the expanding uterus and your growing baby.

If you have experienced miscarriages or first-trimester bleeding, practice only gentle and restorative poses and breath practice (pranayama) during the first trimester, such as:

1. Deep Hip Meditation (see p. 42)

2. Reclining Lower Back Meditation with Ocean Breath

3. Pelvic Tilt

4. Sacral Circles (see p. 92)

5. Reclining Bound Angle Pose

6. Reclining Tree Pose

7. Reclining Crescent Moon Pose

8. Cow-Pose (a) and Child's-Pose (b) Flow

9. Supported Upper Back Stretch

10. Restorative Twist Pose

11. Restorative Cleanser

12. Deep Relaxation Variation 3

Once your pregnancy is firmly established in the second trimester, you can practice the poses listed below, using support whenever your body needs extra comfort.

See next page for photos.

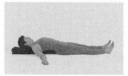

2 (FIG. 4.1)

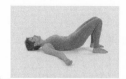

3 (FIG. 2.1)

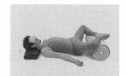

5 (FIG. 2.17)

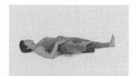

6 (FIG. 3.10)

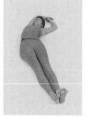

7 (FIG. 4.2)

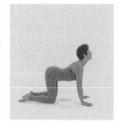

8A (FIG. 2.3)

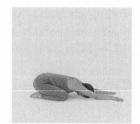

8B (FIG. 2.18)

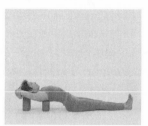

9 (FIG. 6.2)

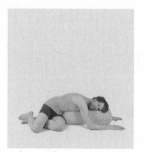

10 (FIG. 3.22)

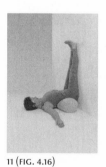

11 (FIG. 4.16)

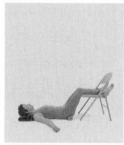

12 (FIG. 4.17)

YOGA FOR A HEALTHY LOWER BACK

Here are some tips for practicing yoga in the second and third trimesters of pregnancy:

- In reclining poses, support your trunk on bolsters and place a folded blanket under your head.
- In standing forward-bending poses, support your hands on blocks or a chair to maintain length along your front torso, and step your feet farther apart from each other.
- Support your body at a wall for fatigue or lower back pain.
- Practice reclining poses and Inverted Cleanser Pose only as long as you are comfortable lying on your back.
- In Child's Pose, support your upper chest and your head on folded blankets or bolsters.
- In Deep Relaxation, lie on your side with a pillow under your head, between your knees, and in front of your chest to support your upper arm.

The following sequence is designed to:

- Increase hip flexibility and tone as preparation for childbirth
- Develop mental and emotional balance through breath practice (pranayama) as an aid to help with mood shifts from hormonal changes
- Strengthen your legs and lower back so your legs can better help you carry your baby without overworking or fatiguing your lower back
- Relieve muscular tightness, fatigue, and pain in your lower back
- Relieve stiffness in your upper back and shoulders
- Encourage good posture, which is important for maintaining lower back health and creating space for your expanding uterus
- Gently massage and stimulate blood flow throughout your abdominal organs and uterus
- Massage your ankles and legs to help to drain extra fluid from your legs
- Rest your legs and hips

1. Seated Bound Angle Pose

2. Wide-Legged Seated Pose

3. Seated Lower Back Side Stretch

4. Cat (a) / Cow (b) Cycle

5. Big Hip Circles

6. Table Balance Pose

7. Deep Hip Bend

8. Noble Warrior Pose

9. Half-Moon Pose

10. Supported Deep Lunge

11. Wide-Legged Standing Forward Bend

12. Reclining Lower Back Meditation with Ocean Breath (use 1 or 2 bolsters to support your trunk; place a thickly folded blanket under your head)

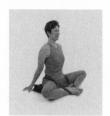
1 (FIG. 2.23)

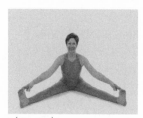
2 (FIG. 2.24)

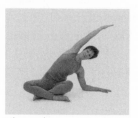
3 (FIG. 4.4)

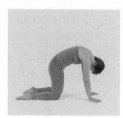
4A (FIG. 2.2)

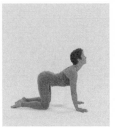 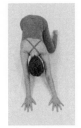 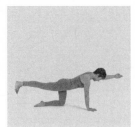 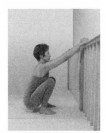

4B (FIG. 2.3)   5 (FIG. 2.4)   6 (FIG. 3.11)   7 (FIG. 2.9)

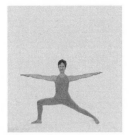 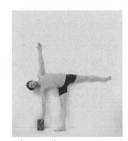 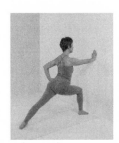 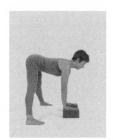

8 (FIG. 2.11)   9 (FIG. 4.11)   10 (FIG. 3.12)   11 (FIG. 3.30)

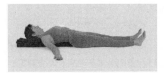

12 (FIG. 4.1)

Notes

Chapter 1: The Journey into Wellness

1. Arthur F. Dalley and Keith L. Moore, *Clinically Oriented Anatomy, Fourth Edition* (Philadelphia: Lippincott Williams & Wilkins, 1999), 432–35.
2. Merriam-Webster Dictionary, "Fascia," www.merriam-webster.com/dictionary/fascia.
3. MedicineNet, "Myo-," www.medterms.com/script/main/art.asp?articlekey=19884.
4. Thomas W. Myers, *Anatomy Trains, Second Edition* (Edinburgh: Elsevier, 2009), 1, 4.
5. Merriam-Webster Dictionary, "Tendon," www.merriam-webster.com/dictionary/tendon.
6. Merriam-Webster Dictionary, "Ligament," www.merriam-webster.com/dictionary/ligament.
7. Medline Plus, "Synovial Fluid," www.nlm.nih.gov/medlineplus/ency/imagepages/19698.htm.
8. Dalley and Moore, 432.
9. *United States Bone and Joint Decade: The Burden of Musculoskeletal Diseases in the United States* (Rosemont, Ill.: American Academy of Orthopaedic Surgeons, 2008), 21.
10. Ibid, 23–24.
11. Ayren Jackson-Cannady, "When to See Your Doctor about Back Pain," www.webmd.com/back-pain/living-with-low-back-pain-11/when-to-call-doctor.
12. Herbert Benson, *The Relaxation Response* (New York: HarperCollins, 1975), 32–33.
13. Jon Kabat-Zinn, *Full Catastrophe Living: Using the Wisdom of Your Body and Mind to Face Stress, Pain, and Illness, 15th Anniversary Edition* (New York: Bantam Dell, 2005), 95.

14. Ibid., 96.
15. R. Saper, et al. "Yoga for Chronic Low Back Pain in a Predominantly Minority Population: A Pilot Randomized Controlled Trial," *Alternative Therapies in Health and Medicine* 15, no. 6 (November–December 2009):18–27.
16. C. C. Streeter, et al. "Effects of Yoga on the Autonomic Nervous System, GABA, and Allostasis in Epilepsy, Depression, and Post-Traumatic Stress Disorder," *Medical Hypotheses* 78, no. 5 (May 2012): 573–74.
17. Yoga Journal, "Yoga in America Market Study 2008," www.yogajournal.com/advertise/press_releases/10.
18. Arvind Sharma, *Our Religions: The Seven World Religions Introduced by Preeminent Scholars from Each Tradition* (San Francisco: Harper SanFrancisco, 1993), 37.
19. Stephen Prothero, *Religious Literacy: What Every American Needs to Know—and Doesn't* (San Francisco: Harper SanFrancisco, 2007), 232.
20. Yoga Journal, "Yoga in America Market Study 2008."
21. Shiva Rae, "You Are Here," www.yogajournal.com/wisdom/460.
22. Edwin F. Bryant, *The Yoga Sutras of Patanjali* (New York: North Point Press, 2009), 3.
23. Ibid., 571.
24. B.K.S. Iyengar, *Light on Pranayama* (New York: Crossroad, 1988), 123.
25. Ben Benjamin, "Unraveling the Mystery of Low Back Pain #1: Sacroiliac Dysfunction," www.benbenjamin.com.
26. DoYoga with Doug Keller, www.doyoga.com.
27. Mary Pullig Schatz, *Back Care Basics* (Berkeley: Rodmell Press, 1992), 47.
28. John J. Triano and Nancy C. Selby, "Ergonomics of the Office and Workplace: An Overview," www.spine-health.com/wellness/ergonomics/ergonomics-office-and-workplace-overview.
29. Iyengar, 233.
30. Philosophico Literary Research Department of Kaivalyadhama S.M.Y.M. Samiti, Lonavla, India, *Yoga Kosha* (New Delhi: Model Press, 1991), 117.
31. *Yoga Journal*, "Yoga in America Market Study 2008."

CHAPTER 2: YOUR HIPS

1. Laura Miller, "Orthopedic Pain Patient Visit Statistics: 4 Areas to Know," http://beckersorthopedicandspine.com/orthopedic-spine-practices-improving-profits/item/3762-orthopedic-pain-patient-visit-statistics-4-areas-to-know.
2. Thomas W. Myers, *Anatomy Trains, Second Edition* (Edinburgh: Elsevier, 2009), 4.
3. Harish Johari, *Chakras: Energy Centers of Transformation* (Rochester, Vt.: Destiny Books, 1987), 55.

4. Guru Prem Singh Khalsa and Harijot Prem Singh Khalsa, *Divine Alignment* (Beverly Hills: Cherdi Kala, Inc., 2003), 3, 15.
5. Edwin F. Bryant. *The Yoga Sutras of Patanjali* (New York: North Point Press, 2009), 283.
6. Doug Keller, "Sacroiliac Support," *Yoga + Joyful Living* (Fall 2009): 62.
7. Ibid., 59.
8. Philosophico Literary Research Department of Kaivalyadhama S.M.Y. M. Samiti, Lonavla, India, *Yoga Kosha* (New Delhi: Model Press, 1991), 324.
9. Georg Feuerstein, *Encyclopedic Dictionary of Yoga* (New York: Paragon House, 1990), 141.
10. T.K.V. Desikachar, *The Heart of Yoga* (Rochester, Vt.: Inner Traditions International, 1995), 175.

CHAPTER 3: YOUR SACRUM

1. Medscape Today, "Anatomy of the Sacrum: Embryology," www.medscape.com/viewarticle/461094_2 (free login required).
2. Diane Lee, *The Pelvic Girdle: An Approach to the Examination and Treatment of the Lumbopelvic-Hip Region, Third Edition* (Edinburgh: Churchill Livingstone, 2004), 60.
3. Harish Johari, *Chakras: Energy Centers of Transformation* (Rochester, Vt.: Destiny Books, 1987), 56.
4. Ibid., 30.
5. Ben Benjamin, "Unraveling the Mystery of Low Back Pain #1: Sacroiliac Dysfunction," www.benbenjamin.com.
6. American Academy of Orthopaedic Surgeons, "Hamstring Muscle Injuries," http://orthoinfo.aaos.org/topic.cfm?topic=a00408.
7. Kevin Durkin, "Pelvic Balancing Sequence," http://kevindurkinyoga.com/Pelvic_Balancing_Sequence.htm.
8. Ibid.
9. Linda Sparrowe and Patricia Walden, *The Women's Book of Yoga & Health* (Boston: Shambhala, 2002), 184.
10. Judith Lasater, *Relax and Renew: Restful Yoga for Stressful Times, Second Edition* (Berkeley: Rodmell Press, 2011), 44–45.
11. Alistair Shearer, *The Yoga Sutras of Patanjali* (New York: Bell Tower, 1982), 95–96.
12. Edwin F. Bryant. *The Yoga Sutras of Patanjali* (New York: North Point Press, 2009), 283.
13. William J. Broad, *The Science of Yoga* (New York: Simon & Schuster, 2012), 95.
14. Judith Lasater, *Yogabody: Anatomy, Kinesiology, and Asana* (Berkeley: Rodmell Press, 2009), 138.

Chapter 4: Your Lumbar Spine

1. *United States Bone and Joint Decade: The Burden of Musculoskeletal Diseases in the United States* (Rosemont, Ill.: American Academy of Orthopaedic Surgeons, 2008), 21.
2. Medline Plus, "Low Back Pain: Acute," www.nlm.nih.gov/medlineplus/ency/article/007425.htm.
3. PubMed Health, "Herniated Disk," www.ncbi.nlm.nih.gov/pubmedhealth/PMH0001478.
4. The Free Dictionary, "Sciatic Nerve," http://medical-dictionary.thefreedictionary.com/sciatic+nerve.
5. Spine-Health, "Radicular Pain and Radiculopathy Definition," www.spine-health.com/glossary/r/radicular-pain-and-radiculopathy. See also University of Maryland Medical Center, "Back Pain and Sciatica: Symptoms and Causes," www.umm.edu/patiented/articles/what_causes_pain_low_back_pain_or_sciatica_000054_2.htm.
6. Medline Plus, "Lordosis," www.nlm.nih.gov/medlineplus/ency/article/003278.htm.
7. Ibid.
8. Vasant L. Lad and Anisha Durve, *Marma Points of Ayurveda: The Energy Pathways for Healing Body, Mind and Consciousness with a Comparison to Traditional Chinese Medicine* (Albuquerque: The Ayurvedic Press, 2008), 19.
9. Ibid., 181.
10. The Free Dictionary, "Sciatic Nerve," http://medical-dictionary.thefreedictionary.com/sciatic+nerve.
11. Marma Points, 180.
12. John E. Sarno, *Healing Back Pain: The Mind-Body Connection* (New York: Warner Books, 1991).
13. Judith Lasater, Ph.D., P.T., *Yogabody: Anatomy, Kinesiology, and Asana* (Berkeley: Rodmell Press, 2009), 138.
14. B.K.S. Iyengar, *Light on Yoga, Revised Edition* (New York: Schocken Books, 1977), 159. See also Yoga Journal, "Marichi's Pose," www.yogajournal.com/poses/691.

Chapter 5: Your Abdominal Core

1. Diane Lee, *The Pelvic Girdle: An Approach to the Examination and Treatment of the Lumbopelvic-Hip Region, Third Edition* (Edinburgh: Churchill Livingstone, 2004), 192.
2. Judith Lasater, Ph.D., P.T., *Yogabody: Anatomy, Kinesiology, and Asana* (Berkeley: Rodmell Press, 2009), 138.
3. C. C. Streeter, et al. "Effects of Yoga on the Autonomic Nervous System, GABA, and Allostasis in Epilepsy, Depression, and Post-Traumatic Stress Disorder," *Medical Hypotheses* 78, no. 5 (May 2012): 571–72.

4. R. P. Brown and P. L. Gerbarg, "Sudarshan Kriya Yogic Breathing in the Treatment of Stress, Anxiety, and Depression: Part I—Neurophysiologic Model," *Journal of Alternative and Complementary Medicine* 11 (2005): 191.

5. Streeter et al., 573–74.

6. R. P. Brown and P. L. Gerbarg, "Sudarshan Kriya Yogic Breathing in the Treatment of Stress, Anxiety, and Depression: Part II—Clinical Applications and Guidelines," *Journal of Alternative and Complementary Medicine* 11 (2005): 711, 714.

7. Edwin F. Bryant. *The Yoga Sutras of Patanjali* (New York: North Point Press, 2009), 35.

8. Vasant L. Lad and Anisha Durve, *Marma Points of Ayurveda: The Energy Pathways for Healing Body, Mind and Consciousness with a Comparison to Traditional Chinese Medicine* (Albuquerque: The Ayurvedic Press, 2008),164–68.

9. Ibid., 69, 313–16

10. Alistair Shearer, *The Yoga Sutras of Patanjali* (New York: Bell Tower, 1982), 102.

11. B.K.S. Iyengar, *Light on the Yoga Sutras of Patanjali* (India: HarperCollins, 1993), 102.

12. Doug Keller, *Yoga as Therapy, Volume Two: Applications* (self-published, 2010), 189–90.

13. B.K.S. Iyengar, *Light on Pranayama* (New York: Crossroad, 1988), 179.

14. Ibid.

15. Harish Johari, *Chakras: Energy Centers of Transformation* (Rochester, Vt.: Destiny Books, 1987), 32–36.

16. Iyengar, *Light on the Yoga Sutras of Patanjali*, 5.

17. Iyengar, *Light on Pranayama*, 97.

18. Angela Tian Zhu, "Dan Tian: Qi Core of Humanity," www.traditionalqi .com/2011/05/24/dan-tian-%E2%80%93-qi-core-of-humanity.

19. Miura Kunio, *The Revival of Qi: Taoist Meditation and Longevity Techniques*, ed. Livia Kohn (Ann Arbor: The University of Michigan Center for Chinese Studies, 1989), 338.

CHAPTER 6: YOUR MIDDLE BACK, UPPER BACK, AND NECK

1. J. Talbot Sellers, "Causes of Upper Back Pain," www.spine-health.com/ conditions/upper-back-pain/causes-upper-back-pain.

2. Sports Injury Clinic, "Tight Muscles in the Upper Back and Neck," www .sportsinjuryclinic.net/sport-injuries/upper-back-neck/tight-muscles-neck.

3. The Free Dictionary, "Vertebral Subluxation Complex," http:// medical-dictionary.thefreedictionary.com/Vertebral+subluxation.

4. Arthur F. Dalley and Keith L. Moore, *Clinically Oriented Anatomy, Fourth Edition* (Philadelphia: Lippincott Williams & Wilkins, 1999), 438.

5. Doug Keller, "Banish Pack Pain," *Yoga + Joyful Living* (March/April 2007): 77.

6. Julie Gudmestad, "Ease on Back," www.yogajournal.com/health/125.

7. http://www.smart-strength-training.com/upper-back-muscles.html.

8. International Olympic Committee, "Factsheet: Records and Metals, Games of the Olympiad," www.olympic.org/Documents/Reference_doc uments_Factsheets/Records_and_medals_at_the_Games_Olympiad.pdf.

9. Keller, 79.

10. Thomas W. Myers, *Anatomy Trains, Second Edition* (Edinburgh: Elsevier, 2009), 164.

11. Ibid., 85.

12. Dalley and Moore, 1001, 1022.

13. Myers, 108–109.

14. Dalley and Moore, 1026.

15. Ibid.

16. Myers, 109.

17. Ibid, 86–87.

18. Edwin F. Bryant. *The Yoga Sutras of Patanjali* (New York: North Point Press, 2009), 364.

19. B.K.S. Iyengar, *Light on the Yoga Sutras of Patanjali* (India: HarperCollins, 1993), 203.

20. Georg Feuerstein, *The Shambhala Encyclopedia of Yoga* (Boston: Shambhala, 1997), 322.

21. Harish Johari, *Chakras: Energy Centers of Transformation* (Rochester, Vt.: Destiny Books, 1987), 139.

22. Ibid., 87.

23. Johari, 149.

24. Feuerstein, 22.

25. Johari, 68.

26. Bryant, 364.

27. Vasant L. Lad and Anisha Durve, *Marma Points of Ayurveda: The Energy Pathways for Healing Body, Mind and Consciousness with a Comparison to Traditional Chinese Medicine* (Albuquerque: The Ayurvedic Press, 2008), 152.

28. Feuerstein, 15, 222.

29. Johari, 63.

30. Feuerstein, 331.

31. Johari, 73.

32. Ibid., 72.

33. Ibid.

34. B.K.S. Iyengar, *Light on Pranayama* (New York: Crossroad, 1988), 272.

35. C. C. Streeter, et al., "Effects of Yoga on the Autonomic Nervous System, GABA, and Allostasis in Epilepsy, Depression, and Post-Traumatic Stress Disorder," *Medical Hypotheses* 78, no. 5 (May 2012): 573–74.

36. Kit Laughlin, *Overcome Neck and Back Pain* (New York: Simon & Schuster, 1995), 82–84.
37. B.K.S. Iyengar, *Light on Yoga, Revised Edition* (New York: Schocken Books, 1977), 251.
38. Alistair Shearer, *The Yoga Sutras of Patanjali* (New York: Bell Tower, 1982), 90.
39. Bryant, 10.
40. Barbara Stoler Miller, *Yoga: Discipline of Freedom* (Berkeley and Los Angeles: University of California Press, 1996), 29.
41. Georg Feuerstein, *The Yoga-Sutra of Patanjali: A New Translation and Commentary* (Rochester: Inner Traditions, 1989), 28.
42. Bryant, 22.
43. Miller, 29.
44. Merriam-Webster Dictionary, "Mandala," www.merriam-webster.com/dictionary/mandala.

Chapter 8: Practices for Specific Lower Back Conditions and Diagnoses

1. WebMD, "Herniated Disc: Topic Overview," www.webmd.com/back-pain/tc/herniated-disc-topic-overview.
2. Loren Fishman and Carol Ardman, *Relief Is in the Stretch* (New York: W. W. Norton & Company, 2005), 90.
3. PubMed Health, "Spinal Stenosis," www.ncbi.nlm.nih.gov/pubmedhealth/PMH0001477.
4. PubMed Health, "Spondylolisthesis," www.ncbi.nlm.nih.gov/pubmedhealth/PMH0002240.
5. PubMed Health, "Fibromyalgia," www.ncbi.nlm.nih.gov/pubmedhealth/PMH0001463.
6. Timothy McCall, *Yoga as Medicine: The Yogic Prescription for Health and Healing* (New York: Bantam Dell, 2007), 301.

Glossary

1. The Sanskrit glossary was compiled in consultation with Benjamin Williams, PhD candidate at Harvard University. In addition, the following books were used:
   Vaman Shivaram Apte, *The Practical Sanskrit-English Dictionary* (New Delhi: Motilal Banarsidass, 1998).
   B.K.S. Iyengar, *Light on Pranayama* (New York: Crossroad, 1988).
   Harish Johari, *Chakras: Energy Centers of Transformation* (Rochester, Vt.: Destiny Books, 1987).

Vasant L. Lad and Anisha Durve, *Marma Points of Ayurveda: The Energy Pathways for Healing Body, Mind and Consciousness with a Comparison to Traditional Chinese Medicine* (Albuquerque: The Ayurvedic Press, 2008).

M. A. Monier-Williams, *Sanskrit-English Dictionary Etymologically and Philologically Arranged with Special Reference to Cognate Indo-European Languages* (Oxford: Clarendon Press, 1899).

Glossary of Sanskrit Terms[1]

AGNI—The element of fire; the fire of transformation; sacrificial fire; the fire of the stomach.

AHIMSA—Nonviolence and noninjury; one of the prerequisite attitudes of a yogi.

AKASHA—Radiance; luminous inner space; the element of ether; sky, atmosphere.

APANA VAYU—Downward, grounding energy located in the lower abdomen; lower wind; lower flow.

ASANA—Posture; physical poses practiced in hatha yoga; the third of Patanjali's eight limbs of yoga; lit. "sitting down; a seat."

AYURVEDA—Holistic system of medicine used in India; lit. "the science of life."

BANDHA—Bond; binding; lock; connection.

- MULA BANDHA—Root Lock; a method of containing energy in the lower pelvis.
- JALANDHARA BANDHA—Chin Lock; a method of containing energy in the neck and upper chest.
- UDDIYANA BANDHA—Abdominal Lock; a method of containing energy in the abdominal cavity.

CHAKRA—One of seven centers of spiritual energy in the body; lit. "wheel, cycle, hollow."

- MULADHARA—The first chakra; root chakra; lit. "root support."
- SVADHISTHANA—The second chakra; sacral chakra; lit. "one's own abode."

- MANIPURA—The third chakra; navel chakra; lit. "city of gems, or jewels."
- ANAHATA—The fourth chakra; heart chakra; lit. "unstruck, unbeaten."
- VISHUDDHA—The fifth chakra; throat chakra; lit. "purity, clarity."
- AJNA—The sixth chakra; third-eye chakra; lit. "command."
- SAHASRARA—The seventh chakra; crown chakra; lit. "thousand-petaled" [lotus].

CHITTA-VISHRANTI—Mental repose.

DHARMA—Nature; characteristics; quality; duty; virtue.

GRANTHI—Knot; tie; hardening; complaint; examples include Brahma, Vishnu, and Rudra.

GUNA—Quality or attribute of nature; see also rajas, tamas, sattva.

IDA—A major energy channel that travels up the spine, crossing with its complement, Pingala, at each chakra; left-hand side; moon; mental force.

KRIYA—Cleansing practice; lit. "action, or activity."

KUMBHA—A water pot, a pitcher, or a chalice.

KUMBHAKA—Breath retention after full inhalation or breath suspension after full exhalation; see also kumbha.

KUNDALINI—Coiled, as in energy; serpentine energy, released through the practice of yoga, which travels up the body's major energy channel; see also Sushumna.

MARMA—The name for the vital energy points on the surface of the body where different aspects of consciousness can be accessed; lit. "hidden."

MUDRA—A symbolic hand gesture used as a meditation aid; a token or mark of divine attributes; lit. "seal, or sign"; derived from *mud*, meaning "to please [the gods]."
- ANJALI MUDRA—The hand gesture of salutation, benediction, or celebration; lit. "offering."
- JNANA MUDRA—The hand gesture of knowledge.
- MANDALA MUDRA—The hand gesture that symbolizes a circle of wholeness; lit. "circular seal."

NABHI CHAKRA—Another name for Manipura chakra; the place from which many of the 72,000 nadis originate; lit. "navel wheel."

NADI—A channel that carries energy throughout the body; see also Ida, Pingala, and Sushumna; from the root *nad*, meaning "to vibrate"; lit. "a river, flowing stream."

Glossary of Sanskrit Terms

NAMASTE—A greeting or salutation, often said at the beginning and/or end of a yoga class, meaning the divine spark within me honors the divine spark within you; lit. "I bow to you."

NISCHALA—Stillness; immovable; a state of serenity; lit. "without movement."

PINGALA—A major energy channel that travels up the spine, crossing with its complement, Ida, at each chakra; right-hand side; sun; positive energy; lit. "yellow or golden."

PRAKASHA—Light; luminosity; brightness; enlightenment; clear radiance; illumination.

PRANA—Life force; vital energy; lit. "breath."

PRANA VAYU—The intake of vital energy; upward, expansive wind, upward flow of energy that resides chiefly in the chest.

PRANAYAMA—Breath-control technique used as an aid to meditation in yoga practice, the fourth of Patanjali's eight limbs of yoga; lit. "restraint of the breath."

- BHASTRIKA PRANAYAMA—Bellows Breath.
- DIRGHA PRANAYAMA—Three-Part Breath; lit. "long or extended breath control."
- KAPALABHATI PRANAYAMA—Shining-Skull Breath.
- UJJAYI PRANAYAMA—Ocean Breath; lit. "upward victory breath control."

RAJAS—Movement; activity; passion; one of the major gunas, or qualities of nature.

SATTVA—Illumination; purity; goodness; one of the major gunas, or qualities of nature.

SHANTI—Peace.

STHIRA—Stable; steadfast, firm; steady.

SUKHAM—Comfort; comfortable; easy; natural; delight; happiness.

SUSHUMNA—The central energy channel of the body, which travels up the spinal column; the path of uncoiled Kundalini energy; see also nadi, Ida, and Pingala.

TAMAS—Inertia; rest; dullness; darkness; one of the major gunas, or qualities of nature.

TAPAS—Purification; self-discipline; heat; austerity.

VAYU—Wind; flow; see also apana vayu and prana vayu.

VINYASA—Movement synchronized with breath; sequential, flowing approach to yoga asana practice; lit. "composition, or arrangement."

YOGA—The discipline of the body, mind, and spirit, using a number of personal practices including physical postures, breathing techniques, and meditation; yoke; union; concentration; path; method; see also asana and pranayama.

Recommended Reading for Lower Back Health

Your journey into wellness doesn't end when you close this book. The books listed below can help deepen your self-knowledge, expand your yoga practice, and generally illuminate your path to lower back health.

ANATOMY, PHYSIOLOGY, AND CHRONIC PAIN:

Benson, Herbert. *The Relaxation Response.* New York: HarperCollins, 1975.

Broad, William J. *The Science of Yoga.* New York: Simon & Schuster, 2012.

Coulter, H. David. *Anatomy of Hatha Yoga: A Manual for Students, Teachers, and Practitioners.* Honesdale, Pa.: Body and Breath, Inc., 2001.

Ellsworth, Abigail. *Anatomy of Yoga: An Instructor's Guide to Improving Your Poses.* Buffalo, N.Y.: Firefly Books, 2010.

Fishman, Loren, and Carol Ardman. *Relief Is in the Stretch: End Back Pain Through Yoga.* New York: W. W. Norton & Company, 2005.

Kabat-Zinn, Jon. *Full Catastrophe Living: Using the Wisdom of Your Body and Mind to Face Stress, Pain, and Illness, 15th Anniversary Edition.* New York: Bantam Dell, 2005.

Koch, Liz. *The Psoas Book, Second Edition.* Felton, Calif.: Guinea Pig Publications, 1997.

Lasater, Judith. *Yogabody: Anatomy, Kinesiology, and Asana.* Berkeley: Rodmell Press, 2009.

Laughlin, Kit. *Overcome Neck and Back Pain.* New York: Simon & Schuster, 1995.

Lee, Diane. *The Pelvic Girdle: An Approach to the Examination and Treatment of the Lumbopelvic-Hip Region, Third Edition*. Edinburgh: Churchill Livingstone, 2004.

Long, Ray. *The Key Muscles of Yoga*. Baldwinsville, N.Y.: Bandha Yoga, 2009.

McCall, Timothy. *Yoga as Medicine: The Yogic Prescription for Health and Healing*. New York: Bantam Dell, 2007.

Meyers, Thomas W. *Anatomy Trains, Second Edition*. Edinburgh: Elsevier, 2009.

Sarno, John E. *Healing Back Pain: The Mind-Body Connection*. New York: Warner Books, 1991.

Schatz, Mary Pullig. *Back Care Basics: A Doctor's Gentle Yoga Program for Back and Neck Pain Relief*. Berkeley: Rodmell Press, 1992.

YOGA AND YOGA PRACTICE:

Desikachar, T.K.V. *The Heart of Yoga: Developing a Personal Practice*. Rochester, Vt.: Inner Traditions International, 1995.

Faulds, Richard, et al. *Kripalu Yoga: A Guide to Practice On and Off the Mat*. New York: Bantam Books, 2006.

Iyengar, B.K.S. *Light on Pranayama*. New York: Crossroad, 1988.

———. *Light on Yoga, Revised Edition*. New York: Schocken Books, 1977.

———. *Yoga: The Path to Holistic Health*. London: Dorling Kindersley, 2001.

Kraftsow, Gary. *Yoga for Wellness*. New York: Penguin/Arkana, 1999.

Lasater, Judith. *Relax and Renew: Restful Yoga for Stressful Times, Second Edition*. Berkeley: Rodmell Press, 2011.

Miller, Elise Browning. *Yoga for Scoliosis*. Palo Alto: Shanti Productions, LLC, 2003.

Rosen, Richard. *The Yoga of Breath: A Step-by-Step Guide to Pranayama*. Boston: Shambhala, 2002.

———. *Pranayama: Beyond the Fundamentals*. Boston: Shambhala, 2006.

Scaravelli, *Vanda. Awakening the Spine*. New York: HarperCollins, 1991.

Schiffmann, Erich. *Yoga: The Spirit and Practice of Moving Into Stillness*. New York: Simon & Schuster, 1996.

Sparrowe, Linda, and Patricia Walden. *The Women's Book of Yoga & Health*. Boston: Shambhala, 2002.

Yee, Rodney, with Nina Zolotov. *Moving Toward Balance: 8 Weeks of Yoga with Rodney Yee.* Emmaus, Pa.: Rodale Press, 2004.

Yoga Spirituality and Philosophy:

Apte, Vaman Shivaram. *The Practical Sanskrit-English Dictionary.* New Delhi: Motilal Banarsidass, 1998.

Bachman, Nicolai. *The Language of Yoga: Complete A to Y Guide to Asana Names, Sanskrit Terms, and Chants.* Boulder: Sounds True, 2004.

Bryant, Edwin F. *The Yoga Sutras of Patanjali.* New York: North Point Press, 2009.

Hartranft, Chip. *The Yoga-Sutra of Patanjali: A New Translation with Commentary.* Boston: Shambhala, 2003.

Johari, Harish. *Chakras: Energy Centers of Transformation.* Rochester, Vt.: Destiny Books, 1987.

Lad, Vasant L., and Anisha Durve. *Marma Points of Ayurveda: The Energy Pathways for Healing Body, Mind and Consciousness with a Comparison to Traditional Chinese Medicine.* Albuquerque: The Ayurvedic Press, 2008.

Lowitz, Leza, and Reema Datta. *Sacred Sanskrit Words for Yoga, Chant, and Meditation.* Berkeley: Stone Bridge Press, 2005.

Miller, Barbara Stoler. *Yoga: Discipline of Freedom: The Yoga Sutra Attributed to Patanjali.* Berkeley and Los Angeles: University of California Press, 1996.

Mitchell, Stephen. *Bhagavad-Gita: A New Translation.* New York: Three Rivers Press, 2000.

Shearer, Alistair. *The Yoga Sutras of Patanjali.* New York: Bell Tower, 1982.

List of Yoga Poses by Chapter

Practice for a Healthy Lumbar Spine

Reclining Spinal Twist	Supta Padangusthasana III
Seated Lower-Back Side Stretch	Parshva Sukhasana
Extended Puppy Pose	Adho Mukha Svanasana Variations
Side Puppy Pose	
Downward-Facing Dog Pose	Adho Mukha Svanasana
Variation 1: Supported Downward-Facing Dog Pose	
Variation 2: Dangling Down-Dog Pose	
Deep Side Stretch Pose	Parshvottanasana Variations
Step 1: Half Deep Side Stretch Pose	
Step 2: Full Deep Side Stretch Pose	
Variation: Open-Heart and Standing Seal	
Half-Moon Pose	Ardha Chandrasana
Flowing Bridge Pose	Setu Bandha Sarvangasana Variation
Flying Locust Pose	Shalabhasana Variation 1
Swimming Locust Pose	Shalabhasana Variation 2
Reclining Bolster Twist	Jathara Parivartanasana Variation 1
Inverted Cleanser Pose	Viparita Karani Variations
Variation 1: Active Cleanser	
Variation 2: Restorative Cleanser	
Deep Relaxation: Experience Your Body's Softness	Shavasana Variation 3

Grow and Progress

Marichi's Seated Twist	Marichyasana I
Revolved Wide-Legged Seated Pose	Parivrtta Upavishta Konasana
Balanced Warrior Pose	Virabhadrasana III
Step 1: Half Balanced Warrior Pose	
Step 2: Full Balanced Warrior Pose	
Variation: Proud Warrior Flow	
Cobra Pose Flow	Bhujangasana Variations
Step 1: Sphinx Pose	
Step 2: Cobra-in-the-Grass Pose	
Step 3: Full Cobra Pose	
Head-to-Knee Pose	Janu Shirsasana
Seated Forward Bend Pose	Paschimottanasana
Child's Pose and Deep Relaxation	Balasana and Shavasana Variation 3

Grow and Progress

Chin Lock	Jalandhara Bandha
Revolved Side-Angle Pose	Parivrtta Parshvakonasana Variation
Revolved Half-Moon Pose	Parivrtta Ardha Chandrasana
Wheel (Upward Bow) Pose	Urdhva Dhanurasana
Child's Pose and Deep Relaxation	Balasana and Shavasana Variation 1